MASSAGE TECHNIQUES

A Case Method Approach

FRANCES M. TAPPAN, B.S., M.A., Ed.D.

Director and Assistant Dean
School of Physical Therapy
University of Connecticut

University Book Exchange
Norman, Oklahoma

First printing, July, 1961
The Macmillan Company, New York
Brett-Macmillan Ltd., Galt, Ontario

Second Printing, January, 1968 University Book Exchange
Third Printing, February, 1969 University Book Exchange
Fourth Printing, December, 1970 University Book Exchange
Fifth Printing, September, 1972 University Book Exchange
Sixth Printing, January, 1973 University Book Exchange
Seventh Printing, August, 1973, University Book Exchange

Printed in the United States of America

Library of Congress catalog card number : 61-6166

MASSAGE TECHNIQUES
A Case Method Approach

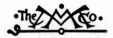

THE MACMILLAN COMPANY
NEW YORK • CHICAGO
DALLAS • ATLANTA • SAN FRANCISCO
LONDON • MANILA

IN CANADA
BRETT-MACMILLAN LTD.
GALT, ONTARIO

MASSAGE TECHNIQUES
A Case Method Approach

The motion picture "Modern Massage Technics" shows all of the basic techniques as described in this text. This 30-minute color film, with sound, can be obtained on loan from the Audio-Visual department of the University of Connecticut, Storrs, Connecticut.

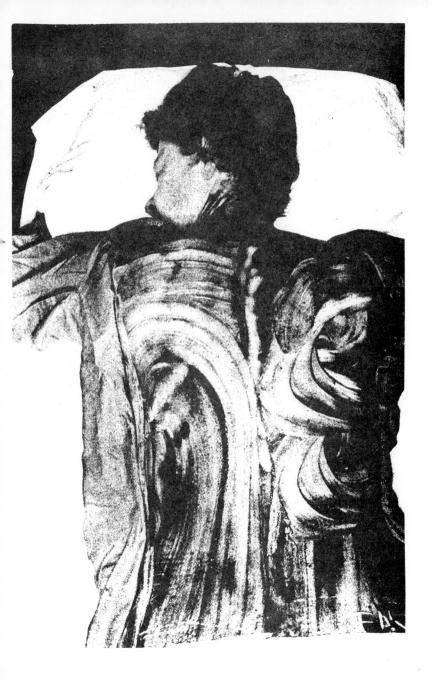

Foreword

This book presents a detailed survey of the variations in the application of massage as practiced in the United States and other parts of the world. Its careful description, comparison, and evaluation of the techniques make it a valuable teaching text. Because of the wealth of reference material presented, it will be an important addition to any library concerned with health and the care of patients.

To provide a complete view of massage techniques, Miss Tappan has included a brief discussion of the work of Elisabeth Dicke. Frau Dicke's system is used widely in Europe, but little attention has been given to it in this country. Research has not yet supported the claims made for Bindegewebsmassage, but the student will be interested in learning its principles and some of the strokes. Some strokes have been adapted by Miss Tappan to fit into systems commonly used in this country.

The case study method as used by Miss Tappan is a standard teaching technique in physical therapy and other fields. However, a word of caution is necessary since there are some examples presented in which massage is contraindicated. The students must be made aware of this.

Each massage system has its own terminology, with strokes common to all systems having several names. As she discusses each system, Miss Tappan has followed its own terminology. This should familiarize the student with the great variety of terms common in massage.

Although a book of this kind is written to aid students, teachers will be pleased to see the work of Albert J. Hoffa, Mary McMillan, and James B. Mennell given well-deserved attention. It is especially interesting to see the influence of Hoffa on techniques presently used in this country.

Miss Tappan's text fills a long-felt need for a book covering all the major systems of massage and giving up-to-date descriptions of the important strokes. The clarity of the illustrations will please both students and teachers.

> John C. Allen, M.D.
> Dean and Medical Director of
>   the School of Physical Therapy
> University of Connecticut

Preface

This text describes the methods of massage currently being used in the United States. Its purpose is to set forth clearly-described and illustrated techniques which students in schools of physical therapy, physical education, nursing, or osteopathy can use.

It is based primarily on the methods of Albert J. Hoffa, Mary McMillan, and James B. Mennell. A complete translation of Hoffa's text, *Technik der Massage,* was made with the help of Miss Ruth Friedlander and these descriptions are included, as well as deviations which have been developed recently. Before the recent deaths of Dr. Mennell and Miss McMillan, I was able to consult with them to assure the accuracy of the descriptions of the methods they used. I am grateful for their interest and assistance.

Elisabeth Dicke's Bindegewebsmassage is discussed. I watched the Dicke techniques as they were taught at the Elisabeth Dicke School in Überlingen, and wrote descriptions of them. These descriptions were rechecked and verified by Gennette Elmeger, a Swiss physical therapist who spoke German and English and studied with Elisabeth Dicke before her death. I take full responsibility for their application here. In some cases reversal of the direction of the stroke has been recommended, and often only part of the total sequence which Dicke prescribed has been included. No claim is made that the reflex effects which Dicke obtained through use of the entire sequence will be obtained by this partial application of some of her techniques.

As a practice guide, a case method is presented, including samples of many of the injuries and illnesses where massage can be usefully applied. This approach leads the student toward solving the problems he will later be faced with. As each student reviews a case, he is expected to relate it to the total care of the patient, applying the general principles which are involved. In so doing, the legal, practical, and psychological aspects of each case should be considered. In planning the massage treatment for these patients, students must be able to see the place of massage in a total treatment plan and not regard it as an isolated method.

The illustrations showing the patterns of the massage strokes were made by applying fingerpaint to the hands of the therapist. The pattern left by powder or other lubricant (which would not show up well in a photograph) is indicated by the fingerpaint pattern. The illustrations show the area covered, as well as the usual patterns, and can guide students as they practice with powder.

F.M.T.

Acknowledgments

It would be humanly impossible to give adequate acknowledgment to all of the many fine people who have contributed to the writing of this book. Primary recognition should be given to Lucille Daniels whose vision and wisdom assisted the author in building a solid foundation in the form of a Master's thesis on massage.

Special gratitude goes to Charles Bollinger of the Macmillan Company. Without his constant encouragement and critical editorial advice, this book would never have been completed.

Josephine A. Dolan, Associate Professor, School of Nursing, University of Connecticut, gave valuable advice concerning the use of massage in the field of nursing.

The members of the staff of the School of Physical Therapy at the University of Connecticut who willingly gave their time, energy, and personal resources deserve credit for their valuable assistance, especially Vera Kaska who used this material for two years and made worthy suggestions which would make this text clearer to those using it for the first time.

The author wishes to thank the following publishers for their permission to quote or summarize from works held in copyright:

Archives of Physical Therapy—for material from "Diagnostic and Therapeutic Massage" (Sept. 1944, Vol. XXV) by Harold D. Storms.

The British Journal of Physical Medicine—for material from "The Usefulness of Massage" (Aug. 1957) by Frances Tappan.

Cassell & Company, Ltd. and Paul B. Hoeber, Inc.—for material from *Treatment by Manipulation and Deep Massage* (1959) by James Cyriax.

J. & A. Churchill Ltd.—for material from *Physical Treatment by Movement, Manipulation and Massage,* 4th ed. (1945) by James B. Mennell.

Ferdinand Enke Verlagsbuchhandlung—for material from *Technik der Massage* (1900) by Albert J. Hoffa.

Hippokrates-Verlag—for material from *Meine Bindegewebsmassage* (1956) by Elisabeth Dicke.

Holt, Rinehart and Winston, Inc.—for material from *The Living Body,* 4th ed. (1958) by Charles H. Best and Norman Burke Taylor.

The Physical Therapy Review—for material from "Massage for the Relief of Pain: Anatomical and Physiological Considerations" (Vol. 40, No. 2, Feb. 1960) by Miriam Jacobs; and material from "Trends in Modern Massage Technics" (Vol. 35, No. 10, Oct. 1955) by Frances Tappan.

W. B. Saunders Company—for material from *Massage and Therapeutic Exercises,* 3rd ed. (1932) by Mary McMillan.

Table of Contents

PART I
General Information

PART II
Techniques Applied

PART III
Variations of Massage Techniques

APPENDIX

1

General Information

I

Introduction

Massage is the systematic and scientific manipulation of the soft tissues of the body. Although massage can be applied by electrical equipment such as vibrators, rollers, or hydrotherapeutic turbines, the purpose of this text is to describe those techniques which can be applied by the hands. Regardless of the individuality developed in the performance of massage, these manipulations will be gliding, percussing, compressing, or vibrating in nature.

Terminology

Common usage of the French terms has named those strokes which glide, *effleurage;* those which knead, *petrissage;* those which strike, *tapotement;* those which compress, *friction;* and those which shake or vibrate, *vibration.*

Purposes of Massage

There are innumerable situations which cause a metabolic imbalance within the soft tissues. Most of these can be treated with massage. The purposes of massage are to bring about any of the physiological, mechanical, or psychological effects attributed to this type of treatment. Through the use of massage, relaxation, relief from pain, reduction of certain types of edema, and increased range of motion can be accomplished. Massage is usually combined with other therapeutic measures, and often provides a form of passive exercise when stretching techniques are used.

There was a time when physical therapy was thought of primarily

2

as heat and massage, combined, to some extent, with exercise. World War II served to bring more emphasis on activity and the exercise program with its newer concept of rehabilitation until the pendulum swung so completely away from passive treatment that massage was seldom prescribed. It is somewhat time consuming, and often the results may seem more psychological than physiological. Even so, realization of the importance of psychology in total patient care should re-emphasize the importance of massage. Massage will not only encourage the confidence of the patient, but will physiologically relieve pain and metabolically prepare the injured or involved muscles to exercise to a greater peak of capacity. The pendulum has now swung toward a sensible combination and massage is once more finding its useful place in the rehabilitation program. The evaluation of the patient's soft tissue, which the therapist can obtain as her hands massage the part, can orient her as no written or verbal report could.

In addition to the treatment of injured or ill people, massage can be used in athletics to ready healthy muscles for strenuous activity, or to assist the body in recovering from the aftereffects of such activity.

The most common uses for massage relate to preparing the musculature and other soft tissue for an exercise program. Therefore, the emphasis of this text will be on the techniques that can accomplish this purpose.

It is the responsibility of those who realize how effectively massage can facilitate rehabilitation to see that patients receive this treatment. If it is not included in the physician's written prescription, often a tactful question will bring the value of massage to his attention.

Massage is a useful and integral part of the physical therapy program. It should be used in its rightful place for psychological, physiological, mechanical, and reflex effects. Long before Christ, and long before it could be explained on a scientific basis, massage was used to relieve pain. A closer look at its history will help to understand the development of massage throughout thousands of years.

2

History of Massage

Massage has been accepted as a therapeutic measure from antiquity. It goes back as far as 2696 B.C., the date of records surviving from Hwang-Ti's description of its use.* In 1800 B.C. the Yoga cult in India used respiratory exercises for religious and healing purposes as recorded in the Veda books of wisdom. Egyptian, Persian, as well as Japanese medical literature, is full of references to bath treatments of various kinds and massage. The ancient Greeks, Herodikos and Hippocrates, have left behind them prescriptions for massage and exercises. In 430 B.C. Hippocrates wrote, "It is necessary to rub the shoulder following reduction of a dislocated shoulder. It is necessary to rub the shoulder gently and smoothly." * They prescribed massage for their patients as well as for their athletes. They established elaborate bathhouses where exercises, massage, and baths were available, but these were patronized by the luxury-loving to the exclusion of the health-seekers. There is in the Pergamon Museum in Berlin a 2000-year-old alabaster relief from the palace of the Assyrian potentate, San Herib, which depicts a massage treatment as realistically as seen in our clinics today.

The pathfinders of ancient medicine were almost forgotten during the Middle Ages. Not until the Sixteenth Century was interest renewed when **Ambroise Paré** sought an anatomical and physiological foundation for mechanotherapy. From then on much, good and bad,

* Walter M. Solomon: "What is Happening to Massage," *Arch. of Phys. Med.,* August, 1950, pp. 521-23.

was written but nothing was actually done for mechanotherapy until the beginning of the last century, when medical gymnastics and massage took on new life through **Per Henrik Ling** of Sweden.

Ling was a fencing master and instructor of gymnastics. He began a study of massage after he had cured himself of rheumatism in the arm by percussions, and developed a method which consisted of massage and medical gymnastics without distinction between the two. It often combined both in a simultaneous application on the theory that massage is a form of passive gymnastics. He based his system on physiology, which was just then emerging as a science.

Through his ardent study and dedication, Ling won acceptance for his new ideas. His method became known as "The Ling System," or "The Swedish Movement Treatment." In 1813 the first college including massage in the curriculum, called the Royal Gymnastic Central Institute, was established in Stockholm at the expense, and under the supervision, of the Swedish government. Ling died in 1839. His students subsequently published his theories, and, through them and the many foreign students at the Central Institute of Stockholm, Ling's system soon became known in a great part of the world.

Reputable institutes of massage and medical gymnastics sprang up in Germany, Austria, and France. People suffering from rheumatism made yearly trips to the spas of Germany and France to take the "cure." This cure consisted of drinking gallons of mineral water, taking mineral baths, graduated exercise, and above all, massage. There was no place in America where one could get the same scientific attention. (This treatment is comparable to our present methods of salicylates, eliminating baths, graduated exercise, and massage.) It was a long time before the medical profession in England and America were willing to consider the matter seriously.

About 1880 **Just Marie Marcellin Lucas-Championnière** claimed that in fractures, the soft tissues as well as bony union should be considered from the start. **Sir William Bennett** of England was impressed with Lucas-Championnière's ideas and started a revolutionary treatment by the use of massage at St. George's Hospital around 1899.

In 1900, **Albert J. Hoffa** published his book *Technik der Massage* in Germany. This book is still the most basic of all texts on massage, giving the clearest description of how to execute the strokes and advocating the procedures that underlie all modern techniques.*

The book by **Max Bohm,** *Massage, Its Principles and Techniques* which was translated by Elizabeth Gould in 1913 also includes some interpretation of Hoffa's techniques.

In 1902, **Dr. Douglas Graham,** a strong advocate of massage, published *A Treatise on Massage, Its History, Mode of Application and Effects.* This text finally aroused the interest of the medical profession in the United States.

Sir Robert Jones, a leading orthopedic surgeon in England and President of the British Orthopedic Association, was an enthusiast for Lucas-Championnière's treatment of fractures. It was with his clinic at Southern Hospital in Liverpool that **Mary McMillan** was associated from 1911 to 1915. In the preface of his book **James B. Mennell** writes, "To Sir Robert Jones I am indebted for the valuable opportunity of working for him at the Special Military Surgical Hospital, Shepherd's Bush: and he has now added to his many kindnesses that of writing the Introduction which follows." † Thus the influence of Lucas-Championnière and Sir Robert Jones was exerted

---

* For the purposes of this study, Hoffa's book was translated for the author by Miss Ruth Friedlander, who was a fellow student at Stanford University. Miss Friedlander was a German student in medicine, and the translation was accomplished by her reading in English as the author took down what she read directly on the typewriter.

† James B. Mennell: *Physical Treatment by Movement, Manipulation and Massage,* 5th ed. The Blakiston Co., Philadelphia (J. A. Churchill, Ltd., London), 1945.

on both Miss McMillan and Dr. Mennell, although neither depends upon the other for the formation of his own system.

In 1917 Dr. E. G. Bracket and Dr. Joel Goldthwait were interested in the reconstruction work that was being done among the allied nations. They were the inaugurators of the Reconstruction Department of the United States Army in the early part of 1918. Short intensive courses were arranged in order to train women to meet the demand. Miss McMillan served as Chief Aide at Walter Reed Army Hospital. It is there that her influence on present techniques was of fundamental importance since, during the last thirty years, a large per cent of our physical therapists have been army trained.

Miss McMillan received her special training in physical therapy in London at the National Hospital for Nervous Diseases, at St. George's Hospital with Sir William Bennett, and at St. Bartholomew's Hospital.

After several years at the Southern Hospital where she was in charge of massage and therapeutic exercise at Greenbank Cripples' Home, she came to the United States as Director of Massage and Medical Gymnastics at Children's Hospital, Portland, Maine. She then took over the responsibility of Chief Aide at Walter Reed Hospital, and Instructor of special war emergency courses of Reed College Clinic for training reconstruction aides in physiotherapy at Portland, Oregon. From 1921 to 1925, when her text was written, she was director of physiotherapy (courses for graduates) at Harvard Medical School.*

James B. Mennell wrote his text, *Physical Treatment by Movement, Manipulation and Massage* in 1917 during World War I. It has been revised several times, the fifth edition appearing in 1945. It is without doubt our most recent reference for massage. As yet few of his suggestions, which tend to break away from the principles that

* Letter from Mary McMillan to Frances Tappan, June 19, 1948.

have been followed for so long, are being used in the field today. In his own words, from the first chapter of this text, he says, ". . . I have had opportunities of watching various workers—English, French, Swedish, Italian, Danish—and have tried to select all that I saw good, and to discard what seemed to me to be bad, in their methods. Thus the views expressed in these pages are founded on the result of many years of close observation, study and experiment. It is possible some of my deductions are erroneous, but at least they are capable of being argued and are not merely arbitrary. The slow but increasing acceptance of many of the principles enunciated lead me now to hope that I may have been able to add something to the advancement of the science and art of physical medicine." [*]

Mennell says in his introduction that he did not intend his book to be used as a text but rather as what he considered the rationale of massage treatment, and an endeavor to show the importance of care and gentleness.

Mennell was the medical officer in charge of physical therapy and lecturer of massage at the Training School of St. Thomas's Hospital, London, England, from 1912 to 1935. Until his death in March, 1957, he worked constantly to interest the medical field in the importance and usefulness of massage.

From 1937 to the present **Gertrude Beard** has contributed to the study of massage through her articles in *The Physical Therapy Review* and through her teaching at Northwestern University. Although none of her writings are directly quoted in this text, many of her concepts have been included.

In addition to her interest in, and contribution to, massage, Miss Beard was president of the American Physical Therapy Association from 1926 to 1928. For many years she directed the School of Physical Therapy at Northwestern University. Through the many gradu-

[*] Mennell, *op. cit.*, p. 2.

ates of this school who had the benefit of her teachings, her influence on massage techniques in America today is profound.

In 1944 **Harold D. Storms** published an article describing a massage stroke which he used both for diagnostic and therapeutic measures, particularly for fibrositic nodules. This technique (described later on pp. 59–60) is still used widely, especially in Canada and Puerto Rico.

Through his book, first published in 1946, **James Cyriax** introduced a specific, limited approach to massage, recommending a type of friction that goes across the fibers of the structure being treated (see p. 60). Because of his excellent illustrations and descriptions, many people in America today use this approach to massage.

In 1929 **Elisabeth Dicke,** a German physical therapist, was suffering from arteriosclerotic changes which involved both lower extremities to the extent that amputation of one leg was considered. While in the hospital awaiting amputation, she managed to massage her own back throughout the night to relieve the severe pain. By morning the circulation was so much better the doctors asked her what she had done. They asked other physical therapists to do the same thing, strictly on a pragmatic basis. If it helped her it would be wise to continue such treatment. The leg improved and amputation was not necessary.

With her curiosity thus piqued, Elisabeth Dicke set upon a sincere study of massage of the lumbar and sacral area in relation to circulation in the legs. She studied the writings of Head and MacKenzie, who describe the relationship between disorders of the viscera and abnormalities of sensation and increased pain in circumscribed areas of the skin. They also describe the relationship of these areas to given segments of the spinal cord. From this information Dicke devised specific massage strokes designed especially to effect specific reflex zones.

This approach emphasizes the importance of knowing exactly

what massage is able to accomplish according to the way it is given, the area covered, the direction of the stroke, and the reflex effects which are possible. It should help those in the profession realize how little we know of the physiological effects of massage and point up the need for effective research in this field.

Summary

Although extensive research needs to be done in order to prove scientifically the effects of massage on the human body, it has been proved pragmatically that massage has been an effective tool for relief of pain through the ages. Perhaps in this scientific era some answers will be found and the true effects of massage will be understood. One factor that makes accurate research difficult is that massage is usually *part* of a total program of rehabilitation. As a *part* we know it can be effective, but to isolate it for research purposes on humans would mean sacrifice of the total program of treatment for the patient. Very little has been done with such animals as mice and dogs. More studies of this type could, and should, be done. Massage is among the oldest forms of treatment, yet it stands in danger of being ignored in an age where it could be understood and effectively used more than ever before. The following discussion of general principles will lay a foundation for such understanding.

3

General Principles of Massage

In order that the student may begin applying massage techniques at once, it will be wise to consider some of the general principles which are basic to all massage.

Ethics

Ethics must be kept in mind at all times. The therapist should have the written order of the doctor and also the patient's complete diagnosis.

Physical contact establishes a close relationship between therapist and patient. This contact should be understanding and sympathetic, but never personal.

Personal appearance

Personal appearance of the therapist should be above reproach. Shoes and uniform should be neat and clean. Name tags assist patients who are not familiar with the hospital personnel. Hair should be neat and worn short or done up so that it does not annoy the patient. Clothing should be comfortable and allow freedom of motion. Short-sleeved uniforms are most practical since they will not drag on the patient, and the cuffs will not become soiled as easily. Because of close contact, the therapist should guard against body or breath odors.

Care of hands

The hands are all important in giving a massage. They should be washed before every treatment. If the patient knows this is done he is then sure that the therapist's hands are clean when they massage him.

Rings should not be worn since they might scratch the patient. The fingernails should be cut so short that the therapist cannot see them if the hands are held up with the palm toward the face.

The hands should always be warm and dry before they touch the patient. If necessary they can be warmed beneath an infrared lamp for a few moments or dried by applying powder to them. They can also be warmed by hot water or by rubbing them briskly together before touching the patient.

Posture

Postural considerations for the therapist will avoid fatigue and backache. In addition, good posture gives a better appearance. The weight should rest evenly on both feet with the body in good postural alignment. If the theapist is massaging a large area, the weight should shift from one foot to the other. A good therapist can apply pressure by a shift of body weight instead of using muscle strength to attain pressure.

Treatment room

The treatment room or booth should at all times be spotless. Linen should be arranged neatly. If the patient sees the therapist put clean linen on the treatment table immediately prior to his treatment, he can be assured that it has been put there for his use only. Linen should be carefully used since laundry is one of a department's greatest expenses, yet all patients should know that their linen is clean.

The temperature of the room should be slightly warmer than normal (about 75°F) since the patient is lying still.

Equipment should be dusted and the metal parts polished. The lubrication containers should be clean and placed within easy reach of the therapist. Containers should not be placed where patients can overturn them.

The treatment table should be the right height to allow for correct postural balance of weight. Obviously, in a department where therapists are of various heights, and each patient presents a different situation, there should be treatment tables of various heights. In addition, a set of platforms ranging from two to six inches in height can be very useful. These platforms should be wide enough and long enough to allow for the complete stance of the therapist, who can place it beside the treatment table if it is found that the patient is too high to be treated comfortably. The therapist should be able to place her hands on the part to be treated without leaning over and without reaching up.

The treatment table should be of wood or metal with a firm pad or mattress, but without springs. Even in the patient's home, ideally the therapist should seek a firm surface, such as a table-top, and not treat the patient in a bed which offers no firm support. There are, of course, numerous exceptions to this ideal. The nurse often gives a back massage to the bed patient.

Positioning the patient

Specific positioning will be discussed with each unit, however there are certain general precautions which should be considered. *Solid support must be given, extending distally and proximally as far as the joints on either side of the injury.*

It cannot be too greatly emphasized that the position should always be one that is comfortable for the patient. There are certain stretching positions that make use of the effect of gravity to put a slight stretch on individual muscles which might need it, but even these should not be so uncomfortable that the patient cannot relax.

In general, the part to be massaged should be elevated in order to allow gravity to assist the mechanical effects of the treatment and make the increased venous return that much easier. Exceptions to this rule will be mentioned later.

At no time should the patient have to exert muscular effort to hold the part being treated in position or to hold the draping about himself. Sometimes sandbags or rolled towels may be used to brace the limb.

Draping

Tight clothing should be removed and a sheet or towel used to cover the parts of the body not being treated. In arranging the draping the patient should not be unnecessarily exposed to the point where it may cause embarrassment. He should be at ease to enjoy his treatment and feel confidence in the person who is about to administer his treatment. Movements of the therapist should be businesslike and should assure the patient that the person giving the treatment is capable and has a professional interest in the problems of the patient.

If the patient is unable to relax because of positioning, lack of adequate support to the part, apprehension concerning his treatment, tight or uncomfortable draping, or discomfort due to being too warm or too cold, the desirable effects of the massage may not be accomplished. Specific positions and basic supportive measures will be discussed later when the massage of each area of the body is described. Although it sounds absurd to mention it, the therapist should never lean on the patient while reaching across the table to arrange the draping.

Lubricants

The *purpose* of a lubricant is simply to avoid uncomfortable friction between the hand of the therapist and the skin of the patient. Older texts may describe shaving the part to be massaged if superfluous hair interferes with the treatment, but such procedure is no longer recommended.

There are many *types of lubricants*. Any lanolin-base cold cream may be used because of its nonirritating qualities. Mineral oil or baby oil may be used as the therapist prefers. Any of the creams or oils can be cleansed from the patient with alcohol. If the primary effect of the massage has been to obtain relaxation, soap and warm water can be used instead of alcohol to remove the lubricant. Care should be taken not to stain the patient's clothes by leaving lubricants on the skin.

When the skin is dry, it is often best *not* to remove the lubricant. In such instances the patient can be advised to wear clothing which can be stained without concern.

When massaging stump ends, 70% alcohol is often used. In these cases stimulation and toughening of the stump is desired.

Some patients might react unfavorably to almost any lubricant. This can usually be eliminated by changing the type of lubricant. Persistent rash should, of course, be called to the attention of the doctor.

Cocoa butter is often used on scar tissue caused by burns or where skin nutrition is indicated, but it has a higher melting point and is, therefore, more inconvenient to use. Olive oil may also be used for skin nutrition, but it becomes rancid quickly and is difficult to keep on hand for general use.

Powder is very useful because it is not so difficult to cleanse following the treatment. An odorless powder should be used, especially for men.

Some therapists prefer to massage with no lubricant, but if this method is used, care must be taken to be sure that the superficial hair of the skin is not pulled and that the hands of the therapist are not moist.

Strong commercial ointments for "rubbing" often produce blisters if used in conjunction with heat and are more irritating to the skin which has been made sensitive by serious illness or injury. Therefore, the use of such ointments is not encouraged. When for psychological reasons the therapist feels that the patient will get more satisfaction from it, such an ointment might be used if there is no pathology or skin condition to contraindicate it. If such stronger ointments have been used by the patient before coming for treatment, care must be taken to wash them off with alcohol prior to administration of any heat or massage.

Too much lubricant prevents a firm contact, and the hands will only slip over the surface of the skin. It would be better to have too little than too much. It remains a common error for many therapists to use lubricants too generously. Many authorities advocate massage without any at all. This author advocates its proper usage and recommends some practice without any in the event this is indicated.

In the early phase of learning massage, tension often causes nervous perspiration of the hands. A solution of alum and alcohol will reduce the amount of moisture and lessen the need for powder.

Pressure and Rhythm

Pressure should be adjusted to the contours of the body and care used over bony areas. All strokes should be rhythmical. The pressure strokes should end with a swing off in a small half circle so that the rhythm will not be broken by an abrupt stop.

Consider the patient's threshold of pain or discomfort. All massage should begin lightly, even in patients who have little involvement or in athletic situations where the person being treated is absolutely normal. As the depth of the stroke increases, the therapist should watch the patient carefully to be sure that pressure is not greater than can be tolerated.

If a muscle tightens under the touch, it has probably been given too severe treatment or so light a touch that it "tickles."

It is important to maintain contact with the patient once the treatment has begun. The hands should not break contact with the skin in deep stroking and kneading except on changing areas. Even though some strokes require an actual loss of contact, the rhythm of the loss should infer that the treatment is a continuing process. Mennell mentions in his description of superficial stroking that the stroke through the air should take the same length of time as the stroke on the body (Mennell, p. 34).

Treatment should not be interrupted. To stop suddenly and adjust the draping, or dry the hands because they have too much lubricant on them, or to turn and talk to someone is upsetting to the patient and to the rhythmical procedure. The telephone should be answered by someone else, unless emergencies arise. In such emergencies the therapist should excuse herself and cover the patient to keep him warm while she is away. Even then the stop should not be sudden, such as lifting the hands in the middle of an effleurage stroke.

Stopping the treatment in order to move around the table or bed to treat the other side should not be done unless both legs, or arms are being treated. Neither should the therapist ask the patient to change position once the treatment has begun. Before the course in massage is completed, students must learn how to approach the patient from almost any angle, since many involvements make it difficult or impossible for the patient to move about easily.

Follow the venous flow
The pressure strokes should be in line with the venous flow, followed by a return stroke without pressure.

Duration
Treatment time is a highly individual decision. Contrary to older texts stating a routine or set time, modern therapists now follow the advice of Mennell and adjust the time to the needs of each patient.

Rest
Rest following treatment is always advised, especially in cases where the involved part is a weight-bearing limb which must be put to work as soon as the patient is ambulatory.

Length of time for this rest must be judged by the therapist If there is swelling in a dependent limb, the resting time should be long enough to permit reduction of swelling before ambulation is attempted.

Summary

If all of these principles are kept in mind the total treatment of massage will proceed more smoothly. They will contribute to the poise of the therapist and establish confidence on the part of the patient. By studying the effects of massage, the therapist will be further able to put the patient's mind at ease through explaining not only *what* is going to be done but also *why* it has been prescribed.

4

Effects of Massage

The effects of massage are mechanical, physiological, reflex, and psychological in nature. By massage, stimulation is provided to the exteroceptors of the skin and proprioceptive receptors of the underlying tissues. Relief of pain is brought about through any one of these effects, or by a combination of any of them.

Mechanical Effects of Massage

Mechanically, massage will assist the venous flow of blood, encourage lymphatic flow, reduce certain types of edema, provide gentle stretching of tissue, and relieve subcutaneous scar tissue.

Assists venous flow

Normally the constant contraction of muscles as people move about pushes against the veins, pressing the blood on toward the heart. When this normal activity is inhibited by injury or illness, the resulting decreased circulation adds another complication to the already disturbed metabolism of the tissues involved.

The mechanical effect of deep stroking on the superficial veins in the direction of the venous flow is easily observed in many persons. The resulting decreased venous pressure provides a favorable situation for an increased arterial circulation. When capillary pressure is reduced, the potentiality for filtration into the extracellular spaces is decreased, thus the load on the lymphatics is also decreased and the possibility of fibrosis is diminished.

Gravity should be considered when possible to assist rather

than inhibit the flow of blood within the veins. The valves within the veins prevent any backflow of blood once it has been encouraged forward. This direct mechanical effect includes mainly the more superficial veins.

Assists lymphatic flow

Lymph is a viscid fluid which moves slowly through the lymphatic system. The lymphatics are, for the most part, noncontractile. Movement of lymph must depend upon outside forces such as the contraction of muscles and pressure generated by filtration of fluid from the capillaries. Immobility due to pain or paralysis seriously interferes with lymph drainage. The lymphatics have a lower pressure and slower flow than the venous flow.

Massage can encourage lymphatic flow, preventing the edema that often occurs with inactivity. Since lymph is viscid and moves slowly, massage strokes should be slow and rhythmical when used for this purpose. Massage is an excellent mechanical substitute when normal muscular function has been interrupted, but active exercise should be encouraged as soon as possible. According to Ladd, Kottke, and Blanchard, massage will increase lymphatic flow, but active exercise will do this more efficiently.

Stretches

Another mechanical effect of massage is the stretching of superficial tissues. When combined with a passive-exercise type of stretching it will encourage the patient to relax and allow further passive stretching of a muscle which has become shortened.

Loosens scar tissue

Subcutaneous scar tissue can at times be loosened by careful and persistent friction. Once it has formed, deeper scarring in connective tissue *cannot* be relieved by massage. Massage can prevent scarring *to some degree* by not allowing stagnation of tissue edema following injury, thus preventing fibrosis.

Physiological Effects

The student of massage should have some understanding of the physiology of the heart and circulation, particularly the peripheral circulation and the return flow of blood and lymph, as taught in basic courses of physiology.

The purpose of this discussion is to summarize and review basic physiology which relates to massage. The extensive readings recommended at the end of this Part will supplement this material.

Metabolism

Metabolically, the muscles maintain a chemical balance through normal activity. As they contract they rid themselves of toxic products by "milking" these acids into the lymphatic and venous flow. As they contract they assist this lymphatic and venous flow toward the heart through mechanical pressure which pushes blood and lymph through channels where valves prevent a backflow. Thus these by-products are carried away.

As the muscles relax, fresh blood flows into them, bringing necessary nutrition to the area.

Overactivity disturbs this balance by not allowing sufficient relaxation time for the inflow of nutritive products. At the same time, due to exertion, toxic products are formed faster than they can be eliminated. Thus the muscle is loaded with irritant acids.

Underactivity also disturbs this balance by not providing the "milking" effect to assist the venous and lymphatic return. Thus the irritant products which form within the muscles are not carried away as they should be and the muscle becomes more or less "stagnant."

Following extreme activity, these irritant acids can be hastened back into the venous return by massage. Often the "lameness" that follows abnormal activity could be lessened or prevented by massage immediately following the activity, since the muscles themselves are inhibited by fatigue.

In many situations, where partial or total muscular inactivity occurs, massage can mechanically assist the "milking" process. However, it can never replace normal muscular activity.

Venostasis

Muscular inactivity can bring about a venostasis, particularly in the dependent limbs where gravity inhibits the normal venous return. Other causes for venostasis may be varicosity, thrombosis, or pressure on the vessels by edema within the surrounding tissues (due to local inflammation or due to the venostasis itself).

It is obvious that massage should *not* be given if there is a possibility of spreading inflammation, if there is a possibility of dislodging a thrombus, thus causing embolism, or if there is such obstruction that the mechanical assistance of massage could not improve the venous flow. Massage given *first* to the proximal aspects of an injured limb will assure the therapist that these circulatory pathways are open enough to carry the venous flow along toward the heart.

Edema

Several causes for edema can be found in *The Living Body* by Best and Taylor. The following is quoted directly from this excellent physiology text:

An increase in the quantity of tissue fluid to the point where it causes a readily detectable increase in volume of a part is called *edema*. It is most frequently seen in the skin and subcutaneous tissues, as a symptom of heart or of kidney disease. When the edema is well marked, the skin appears "puffy" and, when one presses it with a finger, a dent or pit is left which takes a little time to level up again.

Edema is due to an imbalance of those factors regulating the interchange of fluids between the vessels and the tissue spaces. . . . It may result, therefore, from any of the following causes, (a) increased capillary pressure, as in heart disease, (b) reduced plasma osmotic pressure, as in chronic kidney disease, (c) increased permeability of the capillary wall, as in acute kidney disease or as a result of certain poisons, e.g. histamine, (d) obstruction of the lymph channels (lymphatic edema).*

These types of edema should *not* be treated with massage, unless in a specific instance a physician gives careful instructions for an unusual situation.

There are, however, certain types of edema where massage can be of some assistance. Already mentioned is the venostasis caused by muscular inactivity, which may be due to paralysis, injury, or illness. If there is no actual obstruction (such as thrombus) and the edema is caused only by the inactivity of the part there can be no harm in massaging edema from the foot and ankle. An example is a well-healed fracture of the femur which is not yet weight bearing and the leg is allowed to hang down in a dependent position with little or no muscular activity. Without adequate instructions for nonweight-bearing exercises and advice for part-time elevation of the leg (so that gravity can assist the venous return), massage alone will be of little assistance. Massage is not in itself a total treatment but contributes an important part to the total treatment.

In cases of recent injury, where edema is evident due to torn tissues and internal bleeding, massage to the injured area would only encourage further bleeding and more swelling. If massage is indicated at all, it should be given only to areas proximal to the injury, or given so superficially that no further injury would be caused. Massage to any area exhibiting this type of edema should *never* be given until ordered by the physician, who will indicate when sufficient healing has taken place to tolerate such treatment.

Reflex Effects

Recently an active interest has developed in the reflex effects of massage. Sir James MacKenzie defines the reflex process as, "That vital process which is concerned in the reception of a stimulus by

* From *The Living Body*, Fourth Edition, by Charles Herbert Best and Norman Burke Taylor. Reprinted by permission of Holt, Rinehart and Winston, Inc., Copyright 1958, pp. 101–2.

one organ or tissue and its conduction to another organ, which on receiving a stimulus produces the effect." * In massage the hands stimulate the sensory receptors of the skin and subcutaneous tissues, causing reflex effects. The stimuli pass along the afferent fibers of the peripheral nervous system to the spinal cord; from there, it is conceivable that these stimuli may disperse through the central and autonomic nervous systems, producing various effects in any zone supplied from the same segment of the spinal cord. Some of these effects are capillary vasodilatation or constriction, relaxation or stimulation of voluntary muscle contraction, and gooseflesh. In addition, there is the possible sedation or stimulation of sensory reception with sedation or stimulation of pain. In extreme cases reflex effects may be severe. They could cause nausea, vomiting, and depression of the heart's action with resulting pallor and sweating.

On this principle Elisabeth Dicke organized the specific routine described in her text, *Meine Bindegewebsmassage*. If these viscerocutaneous effects are possible it can be seen that beneficial effects from massage of specific zones could be produced with controlled results.

Miriam Jacobs discussed the reflex effects of massage as follows: †

The increased circulation by way of improved superficial venous and lymphatic flow is an effect of deep pressure produced by stroking or compression movements. Mechanical pressure from stroking movements probably also produces direct effects upon the capillaries resulting in capillary contraction as seen in the "white" reaction following mechanical stimulation of the skin. It is said to be of capillary origin and is not dependent upon nerves. According to the standard physiology texts, it may be a direct response of the capillaries to irritation or to some substance

* J. MacKenzie: *Angina Pectoris*. Henry Frowde and Hodder and Stoughton, London, 1923, p. 47.

† Miriam Jacobs: "Massage for the Relief of Pain: Anatomical and Physiological Considerations," *Phys. Therapy Rev.*, Vol. 40, No. 2, (Feb.) 1960, pp. 96–97. Reprinted with the kind permission of Miriam Jacobs and *The Physical Therapy Review*.

triple response

liberated as a result of the mechanical stimulus. With firmer pressure, a "red" reaction appears. This is the result of capillary dilatation and is not dependent upon nervous mechanisms. Stronger stimuli or repeated stimuli produce a "red flare" and is due to dilatation of the arteriole. It is thought that dilatation of the arteriole may be due to a local axon reflex mechanism (1). With an intense stimulus (which is not considered a desirable massage procedure in this country) a wheal may be formed. This "triple response" red reaction, red flare and wheal formation is believed to be brought about by a diffusion of a substance liberated by the cells of the skin in response to mechanical stimulation. The substance bears a resemblance to histamine in its effects; capillary dilatation by its direct effects, arteriole dilatation by the axon reflex, and finally a wheal due to the increased capillary permeability and the release of fluid.

The existence of vasoconstrictor nerve fibers which increase the tone of the arterioles is unquestioned. Their cells of origin are located in the intermediolateral column of gray matter of the thoracic and upper lumbar cord and their fibers pass via the anterior roots to synapse in the chain ganglia via the white rami; they rejoin the segmental spinal nerves via the gray rami to be distributed to the vessels of the skin and muscles. The anatomy of the vasodilator fibers is confusing and debatable. The vasoconstrictor fibers are limited for the most part to the sympathetic system; the vasodilator fibers may not be restricted to the parasympathetic system as is often described. Barron suggests that vasodilator fibers are distributed not only via the parasympathetic outflow but they are also found co-mingled with the vasoconstrictor fibers of the sympathetic outflow (2). Another group of vasodilator fibers are said to be intermingled with the afferents of the spinal nerves. At the periphery, an afferent fiber from a receptor in the skin may give off a collateral to the arterioles of the vascular bed of the skin. Thus, local stimulation of the skin sets up (in addition to the afferent impulses to the central nervous system) an axon reflex that acts upon the arterioles. That vasodilatation does follow experimentally produced antidromic stimulation (causing impulses to flow back to the receptor) of the dorsal root is generally accepted. The question that is debated is whether impulses are normally set up in the central ends of the dorsal root afferents, for neural control of the blood vessels of the skin. Such an antidromic effect could explain the effects of massage; i.e., peripheral stimulation of the sensory afferents resulting in reflex dilatation of the arterioles of the muscles and vascular bed of the skin.

Bayliss has shown that stimulation of the sensory afferent nerves from the limbs in animals brings about vasodilatation due to inhibition of the local vasoconstrictors as well as excitation of the local vasodilators, an effect comparable to reciprocal innervation seen in skeletal muscle (2).

Thus the blood supply increased by the sensory stimulation of massage may be a combination of excitation of the vasodilators and inhibition of the vasoconstrictors.

Barron suggests that evidence is also accumulating which indicates that there are pressure sensitive fibers intermingled in other nerves of the blood vessels of the skin and viscera which if activated bring about a fall in blood pressure through vasodilatation of the splanchnic region (2). He further states that stimulation of the sciatic or other mixed nerves by cooling, activation by weak stimuli or mechanical stimuli may cause vasodilation of the splanchnic area (2). This might explain some of the visceral effects claimed by the advocates of Bindegewebsmassage which may be termed a weak stimulus (3).

Deep pain following ischemia resulting from sustained muscle contraction may be relieved by massage through the improved circulation afforded by, 1) the mechanical pressure on superficial venous and lymphatic channels, and 2) reflex dilatation through stimulation of the cutaneous afferents mediating touch and pressure. Another possibility for the relief of pain may be mediated through another mechanism. The stretch or tension, placed on the tendons and fascia surrounding the muscles during the stretching and compression movements, as in petrissage, may have an inhibitory effect on sustained muscle contraction. It is a well known fact that a "cramped muscle" can be relaxed by stretching it or by deep kneading. Impulses from the tendon sensory organs (probably Golgi tendon organs) and perhaps also from the fascia and adjacent joint structures, which are activated by stretch, produce powerful central inhibition of the neurons controlling that muscle. This effect has been called the inverse myotatic reflex (4). Relaxation and the relief of pain of sustained muscle contraction by massage and traction might possibly be explained on this basis.

(References for Miss Jacobs' Article)

1. Bard, Phillip, *Medical Physiology.* C. V. Mosby Co., St. Louis, 1956, pp. 158–59.

2. Barron, D. J., "Physiology of the Organs of Circulation of the Blood and Lymph." Sec. VI in *Textbook of Physiology,* edited by J. F. Fulton. W. B. Saunders Co., Philadelphia, 1955, pp. 566–87, 755–94.

3. Ebner, M., "Peripheral circulatory disturbances: treatment by massage of connective tissues in reflex zones," *Brit. J. Phys. Med.,* Vol. 19, August, 1956, pp. 176–80.

4. Lloyd, D. P. C., "Principles of Nervous Activity." Sec. I, in *Textbook of Physiology,* edited by J. E. Fulton. W. B. Saunders Co., 1955, pp. 104–9.

Effects of Massage on the Skin

Since the hands contact the skin when massage is done the effects of this treatment on the skin should be considered. One of the major effects is the contact this pressure makes with the sensory nerve endings. Usually massage is sedative and these effects are therefore beneficial. If, however, there is a nerve injury present which makes these sensory nerve endings extremely hypersensitive, so sensitive in fact that massage does not bring sedation but only increases the pain of the patient, it is then contraindicated. It would not be given unless the therapist could lower the pain threshold of the patient by an extremely technical approach. Occasionally these patients can tolerate a firm contact better than a superficial one, and if such were the case, continued massage might be indicated.

The condition of the skin following extreme injury is often abnormal. Parts which have been in a cast will have layers of dead skin under which tender, new skin has developed. In cases where the skin has been burned, massage would not be indicated until adequate scar tissue has formed. Decision as to when this type of tissue may be treated (and it may be a skin graft) is made by the physician in charge.

Because the skin helps remove excretory products its pores must be kept open. The friction of massage will create heat which invites perspiration, and increases sebaceous excretions. The skin also carries out a certain amount of respiration (exchanging carbon dioxide and oxygen) and can be assisted by massage after the part has been in a cast and the normal function of the skin has been inhibited. Massage in these cases helps the skin return to normal function.

If there are layers of dead skin inhibiting the normal functions of skin, they can best be removed by first subjecting the part to whirlpool, followed by massage.

Occasionally a patient's skin will react to massage by breaking out or showing infections of the hair follicles. In the presence of such infections massage is discontinued until reordered by the physician, or the type of lubricant is changed, or occasionally massage with no lubricant at all is given.

Results of Recent Research

Research to determine the physiological effects of massage has disproved some of the theories that have been held. More research needs to be done in this field to prove or disprove some of our present concepts.

Obesity

The old idea that obesity can be reduced by massage has been dispelled. Massage too traumatic for humans to tolerate might bruise the adipose tissue, necessitating replacement with new tissue. However, this new tissue would only be *more* adipose tissue. As a "come on" in reducing salons, massage is combined with steam baths which reduce the water content of the body through excessive perspiration, thus showing an immediate loss of weight on the salon scale. Massage can only induce a psychological feeling of well-being for such customers.

Muscle-mass, strength, and motion

Massage is ineffective in delaying loss of mass and strength following nerve injuries. It will not hasten the recovery of sensation, nor will it produce a better histologic picture. It will, however, accelerate voluntary and reflex action once the nerve injury has begun to recover and re-enervation is present. In such cases massage should be combined with passive and active re-educational exercise.

Therefore, massage is a part of the patient's total rehabilitation program, not an independent treatment to be used by itself. The evaluation of usefulness of massage must consider its role in total patient care.

Total blood flow

Massage does not increase total blood flow nor influence total body metabolism unless it is too traumatic to be tolerated by an individual with an abnormality. After very deep stroking there is some increase in blood flow of the massaged extremity but no change in the contralateral extremity.

Lymph

Massage will increase the flow of lymph to a greater extent than passive motion or electrical stimulation, but at no time can massage adequately substitute for active exercise. This does not mean that the patient requires no massage if he is able to do active exercise. Often, through the sedative effects of massage, *better* active exercise can be accomplished.

Summary

In summary it can be said that massage will increase venous and lymphatic flow; reduce certain types of edema; provide stretching of tissue; relieve subcutaneous scar tissue; improve nutrition through the skin by the application of special lubricants; increase perspiration, thus removing excretory products; help to remove dry scaly skin following casting and assist soft tissue toward normal metabolic balance. In addition to this, there are reflex effects from the stimulation of sensory receptors of the skin and subcutaneous tissues.

Explaining the purpose of the treatment to the patient will strengthen the relationship between therapist and patient. A study of other ways to strengthen these relationships will enable both therapist and patient to work together toward the common goal they mutually share.

5

Patient-Therapist Relationships

Students of massage will realize the importance of understanding the patient's problems, particularly those which arise from his immediate physical deficiencies. The therapist must also understand her own individual personality as much as possible. If she can recognize, for instance, that the patient is compensating or rationalizing, she will find it much easier to laugh at many of the frustrating situations that arise.

The patient

The patient is of primary importance. He is an individual who has developed a personality from the day he was born. He is normal in most respects but faced at the moment with a problem. There has been no one like him before, and there will be no one like him in the future. His reactions to his present environment will logically follow the pattern of his basic personality, although, depending on the severity of his illness or injury, he will be more vulnerable than in a normal situation.

Defense mechanisms

He may meet his problem rationally or resort to mechanisms of defense, such as sublimation, condensation, conversion, repression, projection, identification, compensation, symbolism, displacement, or rationalization.

Most patients are normal individuals

Most individuals will not reach these extremes of emotional reaction, but will react between the extremes. They will recognize their present incapacities and want as much assistance or consideration as is necessary, but no more.

Since the picture people form of themselves as "Selves" is largely determined by the picture they believe others have of them, they like to put their best foot forward and try to react to all situations as normally as possible (Pinter, Eisenson, and Stanton, Chapter I). This premise relates as much to the therapist as it does to the patient. Therefore let it be re-emphasized that the maladjusted behavior exhibited by the patient *is not peculiar just to him*. It is similar to the maladjusted behavior of nondisabled people. It is the same maladjusted behavior the patient may have shown before the physical disability.

It cannot be said that all athletes who are knocked out of a game with an injury will become angry. One boy might be really grateful and relieved that he does not have to struggle any longer with the contest, and the next boy might be truly angry at himself, the coach, or someone on the opposite team who caused him to be put out of the game.

Neither can it be said that *all* people who find themselves severely handicapped will resort to utter despair, despondency, or dependency. According to their usual way of reacting to life's situations, they might be angry, resentful, dejected, apprehensive, or fearful. They may possibly fight these apprehensions with such vigor that the vigor becomes cause for concern.

Normal reaction

One must never lose sight of the fact that a certain amount of reaction is justified and falls well within the range of normalcy. However, the justified anger and sense of frustration of the athlete put out of a game with a minor injury *should* be fleeting, while we would expect the emotional reaction of the one who finds himself severely handicapped for life and unable to support his family to be more lasting. Only if these reactions seem extreme and unwarranted would they cause concern. Depth of expected reaction can be judged only if *all* the facts of the case are known. It is important to know as much about the patient as possible, for it is absolutely impossible to understand his situation otherwise.

If the patient feels extremely helpless, and his personality is such that he objects to this feeling of helplessness, he may reject treatment, such as massage, which makes him feel even more dependent and helpless. The next patient might react with extreme craving for sympathy or employ sympathy-getting methods.

What is most apparent at first is not in all instances a true picture of the individual's reaction. A patient may feel extremely helpless and want attention and sympathy, but at the same time may be ashamed of these emotions and put on a show of *not* wanting attention. This complicates the therapist's attempt to understand and often she will need professional assistance from the psychologist or psychiatrist.

If a given reaction can be recognized as a defense mechanism and not, for instance, an intentional desire on the part of the patient to antagonize, the therapist can with all sincerity maintain her attitude of friendly understanding, often in the face of rather great odds.

Exaggerated reactions

Antagonistic feelings on the part of the patient are not uncommon and are not necessarily the fault of the therapist. The patient may project the helplessness and frustration he feels into antagonistic feelings toward the therapist. Another patient, instead of feeling antagonistic, might worship his therapist or fancy that he has fallen in love with her. Between these two extremes are found the reactions of most patients, who appreciate the fact that someone is trying to help them and sincerely want to cooperate with the program.

It is interesting to point out that even the experienced therapist tends to believe the patients who admire her, thinking, "I guess I'm pretty good." But if the patient is antagonistic she will deny that his antagonism may be based on a fault of her own personality, thinking with true good nature (which is indeed advocated), "Oh well, he must be just projecting his antagonism onto me." This is because therapists are as human as patients and also want to maintain their own ego. True evaluation of one's self is perhaps the most difficult part in a sincere attempt to establish rapport.

Importance of treatment to the patient

The importance of the treatment to the patient can never be over-estimated. Suppose, for instance, that the therapist finds a fibrositic nodule in the upper trapezius of a somewhat neurotic patient. To the therapist this is a matter of interest but not of life and death. The patient may have read in the newspaper that any unexplained lumps should be reported immediately to a physician, since they may be malignant. He feels the lump under the hands of the therapist and immediately wonders if he has cancer. This example may sound extreme but it is not outside the realm of possibility. The first warning to the therapist might be a sweating or paleness of the patient. Even though the patient says nothing of his *apprehension*, the therapist should notice his condition and attempt to find out what has caused this sudden and unexpected reaction.

Reassure and support the patient

The patient can be reassured by explaining every part of his treatment to him and also by giving him an idea of what it is expected to accomplish. If the treatment is designed to help him relax, he can then cooperate by trying to relax.

The nurse can help her patient relax and drop off to sleep by massage, and a few soothing words of explanation as to how the massage will aid the patient in his own attempts to relax.

On the other hand, the athletic coach, who is trying to stimulate a member of his team, can inspire him to greater effort by explaining that this type of massage will put his muscles in the best possible condition for maximum activity.

The patient usually favors the therapist who treated him first, unless some unfortunate circumstances altered this pattern. It is wiser, therefore, to have the same therapist work with a patient so the treatment will remain constant and the two will become acquainted.

Warning signals

As the therapist gains in experience she will learn to recognize the warning signals that indicate antagonism, overaffection, *apprehension,* pain, or other undesirable emotional reactions which might necessitate a change in therapists or technique.

Some patients might prefer a male therapist; others might get along much better with a female. This preference might be due to the type of treatment necessary, or the patient's personality or complexes. Even the experienced therapist can arouse unexpected reactions. It is up to the therapist to watch for warnings that indicate the patient is reacting emotionally to the situation.

There may be blushing or blanching, goose pimples, shortness of breath, sudden tenseness of muscles following a technique or remark, or sudden tears in the eyes. The patient may look away or avoid the eyes of the therapist. He may also stare impudently. He may begin to squirm about or nervously pull away from the treatment. At the very first sign of discomfort, it is up to the therapist to discover whether the patient is apprehensive, embarrassed, or actually uncomfortable. The next step, of course, is to do something to alleviate the situation, even if this means terminating the treatment for the present.

All of the factors relating to personal appearance and cleanliness mentioned earlier cannot be ignored when discussing patient-therapist relationships. A therapist must *look* pleasant, *feel* pleasant, and *be* pleasant at all times.

Empathy

An empathic approach is imperative. It will let the patient know, not so much by what is said or done, but in the way it is said and done, that the therapist *really cares* about the total welfare of the patient. This can be done without pity, or overindulgent sympathy, but with sincere interest in the personal goals and values of each patient.

Summary

In summary then, each therapist must try to understand herself as well as the patient. It is the responsibility of the therapist to make the initial adjustments and work toward the best approach to be used with each patient. The therapist must understand the basic fundamentals of psychology for the handicapped person and the defense mechanisms that most often are used. He must also recognize how much deviation from the normal can be expected for the individual in his present circumstances. It is the responsibility of the therapist to support and reassure the patient and inspire him to cooperate in the program for his total rehabilitation.

Part II of this text will deal with the application of massage techniques. Most students will practice on other healthy students in learning to massage. This should not prevent them from training their hands to locate abnormalities for they will be able to find areas of tension and tightness caused by extensive typing, uncomfortable reading positions, or other student activities causing muscular tension. They will even find that working with each other requires a certain amount of psychological adjustment.

Recommended Readings for Part I

Alexander, R. S.: "The Physiology and Measurement of Peripheral Circulation," *Phys. Therapy Rev.*, Vol. 30, No. 11, (Nov.) 1950, pp. 452–61.

Bard, P.: *Medical Physiology.* C. V. Mosby Co., St. Louis, 1956.

Barker, R. C.; Wright, B. A.; and Gonick, M. R.: *Adjustment to Physical Handicap and Illness.* Social Science Research Council, New York, Bulletin No. 55, 1946.

Barron, D. J.: "Physiology of the Organs of Circulation of the Blood and Lymph," Sec. VI in *Textbook of Physiology* (edited by J. F. Fulton). W. B. Saunders Co., Philadelphia, 1955.

Beard, G.: "A History of Massage Technic," *Phys. Therapy Rev.*, Vol. 32, No. 12, (Dec.) 1952, pp. 613–14.

Best, C. H., and Taylor, N. B.: *The Living Body*, 4th ed. Holt, Rinehart and Winston, Inc., New York, 1958.

Blasko, J. J.: "Some Psychiatric Aspects in a Physical Therapy Program," *Phys. Therapy Rev.*, Vol. 31, No. 11, (Nov.) 1951, pp. 468–73.

Carrier, E. B.: "Determination of Plasma and Hemoglobin Volumes after Unit Hemorrhages under Controlled Experimental Conditions," *J. A. Physiol.*, Vol. 61, No. 528, 1922.

Chor, H.; Cleveland, D.; Davenport, H. A.; Dolkart, R. A.; and Beard, G.: "Atrophy and Regeneration of the Gastrocnemius-Soleus Muscles," *J.A.M.A.*, Vol. 113, No. 1029, (Sept.) 1939.

Copestake, B. M. G.: *The Theory and Practice of Massage*, 4th ed. Paul B. Hoeber, Inc., New York, 1926.

Cyriax, J.: *Treatment by Manipulation and Deep Massage*, 6th ed. Paul B. Hoeber, Inc., New York, Cassell & Company Ltd., London, 1959.

Dicke, E.: *Meine Bindegewebsmassage.* Hippokrates-Verlag, Stutt-
    gart, 1954.
Ebel, A., and Wisham, L.: "Effect of Massage on Muscle Tempera-
    ture and Radiosodium Clearance," *Arch. Phys. Med.,* Vol. 33,
    No. 7, (July) 1952, pp. 399–405.
Ebner, M.: "Peripheral Circulatory Disturbances: Treatment by
    Massage of Connective Tissue Reflex Zones," *Brit. J. Phys.
    Med.,* Vol. 19, (Aug.) 1956, pp. 176–80.
Elkins, E. C.; Herrick, J. F.; Graindlay, J. H.; Mann, F. C.; and
    DeForest, R. E.: "Effect of Various Procedures on the Flow of
    Lymph," *Arch. Phys. Med.,* Vol. 34, No. 1, (Jan.) 1953, pp.
    81–89.
Fulton, J. F.: *A Text Book of Physiology,* 16th ed. W. B. Saunders
    Co., Philadelphia, 1959.
Gammon, G. D., and Starr, I.: "Studies on the Relief of Pain by
    Counter-irritation," *J. Clin. Invest.,* Vol. 20, No. 13, (Jan.) 1941.
Garrett, J. F.: *Psychological Aspects of Physical Disability.* Wash-
    ington, D. C., U. S. Government Printing Office, Rehabilitation
    Service Series, No. 210, 1946.
Graham, D.: *Massage, Manual Treatment, and Remedial Move-
    ments,* 4th ed. J. B. Lippincott Co., 1913.
Head, Sir Henry: *Studies in Neurology.* Henry Frowde and Hodder
    and Stoughton, London, 1920.
Hertzman, A.: "The Physiology and Measurement of Circulation,"
    Phys. Therapy Rev., Vol. 30, No. 11, (Nov.) 1950, pp. 471–81.
Hoffa, A. J.: *Technik der Massage.* F. Enke, Stuttgart, Germany,
    1900.
Jacobs, M.: "Massage for the Relief of Pain: Anatomical and Physio-
    logical Considerations," *Phys. Therapy Rev.,* Vol. 40, No. 2,
    (Feb.) 1960, pp. 96–97.
Karnosh, L. J., and Mereness, D.: *Psychiatry for Nurses.* C. V.
    Mosby Co., St. Louis, 1944.
Kelly, H. T.: "Psychosomatic Aspects of Physical Medicine," *Phys.
    Therapy Rev.,* Vol. 28, No. 6, (Nov.–Dec.) 1948, pp. 280–83.
Kimber, D. C.; Gray, C. E.; Stackpole, C. E.; Leavell, L. C.: *Text-
    book of Anatomy and Physiology,* 14th ed. The Macmillan
    Company, New York, 1961.
Kleen, E. H. G.: *Massage and Medical Gymnastics,* 2nd ed. Wil-
    liams and Wood Co., Philadelphia, 1921.

Kosman, A. J.; Wood, E. C.; and Osborn, S. L.: "The Effect of Massage upon the Skeletal Muscle of the Dog," *Arch. Phys. Med.*, Vol. XXIX, No. 8, (Aug.) 1948, pp. 489–90.

Ladd, M. P.; Kottke, F. J.; and Blanchard, R. S.: "Studies of the Effect of Massage on the Flow of Lymph from the Foreleg of the Dog," *Arch. Phys. Med.*, Vol. XXXIII, No. 10, (Oct.) 1952, pp. 604–12.

Lloyd, D. P. C.: "Principles of Nervous Activity," Sec. I in *Textbook of Physiology* (edited by J. F. Fulton). W. B. Saunders Co., Philadelphia, 1955.

Ludwig, A. O.: "Emotional Factors in Rheumatoid Arthritis," *Phys. Therapy Rev.*, Vol. 29, No. 8, (Aug.) 1949, pp. 339–44.

MacKenzie, J.: *Angina Pectoris.* Henry Frowde and Hodder and Stoughton, London, 1923.

Martin, G., et al.: "Cutaneous Temperature of the Extremities of Normal Subjects and of Patients with Rheumatoid Arthritis: Part III. Effect of Massage on Peripheral Circulation of the Extremities," *Arch. Phys. Med.*, Vol. 27, No. 11, (Nov.) 1946, pp. 665–82.

Maslow, A. H., and Mittlemann, B.: *Principles of Abnormal Psychology.* Harper & Brothers, New York, 1941.

McMillan, M.: *Massage and Therapeutic Exercise*, 3rd ed. W. B. Saunders Co., Philadelphia, 1932.

Mennell, J. B.: *Physical Treatment by Movement, Manipulation and Massage*, 4th ed. The Blakiston Co., Philadelphia, J. & A. Churchill Ltd., London, 1940.

Nissen, H.: *Practical Massage and Corrective Exercises.* F. A. Davis Co., Philadelphia, 1939.

Pemberton, R.: "The Physiological Influence of Massage," in *Principles and Practice of Physical Therapy*, Vol. I. W. F. Prior Co., Inc., 1937.

Pinter, R.; Eisenson, J.; and Stanton, M.: *The Psychology of the Physically Handicapped.* F. S. Crofts & Co., New York, 1941.

Pollock, L. J., et al.: "The Effect of Massage and Passive Movement upon the Residuals of Experimentally Produced Section of the Sciatic Nerves of the Cat," *Arch. Phys. Med.*, Vol. XXXI, No. 5, (May) 1950, pp. 265–76.

Scull, C. W.: "Massage—Physiologic Basis," *Arch. Phys. Med.*, Vol. 26, No. 3, (Mar.) 1945, pp. 159–67.

Smith, L. E.: "Role of Physical Therapy in Care of Psychiatric Patients," *Phys. Therapy Rev.*, Vol. 31, No. 4, (Apr.) 1951, pp. 123–26.

Solomon, W. M.: "What Is Happening to Massage?," *Arch. Phys. Med.*, Vol. 31, (Aug.) 1950, pp. 521–33.

Storms, H. D.: "Diagnostic and Therapeutic Massage," *Arch. Phys. Med.*, Vol. XXV, (Sept.) 1944, pp. 550–52.

Suskind, M. I.; Hajek, N. M.; and Hine, H. M.: "Effects of Massage on Denervated Skeletal Muscle," *Arch. Phys. Med.*, Vol. 27, No. 133, (Mar.) 1946.

von Werssowetz, O. F.: "Psychiatric Rehabilitation of Brachialgia," *Phys. Therapy Rev.*, Vol. 32, No. 4, (Apr.) 1952, pp. 163–69.

Wakim, K. G., et al.: "The Effects of Massage on the Circulation in Normal and Paralyzed Extremities," *Arch. Phys. Med.*, Vol. XXX, (Mar.) 1949, pp. 135–44.

Wood, E.; Kosman, A. J.; and Osborne, S. L.: "Effects of Massage in Delaying Atrophy in Denervated Skeletal Muscle of the Dog," *Phys. Therapy Rev.*, Vol. 28, No. 6, (Nov.–Dec.) 1948, pp. 284–85.

Zausmer, E.: "Psychological Implications in Poliomyelitis," *Phys. Therapy Rev.*, Vol. 30, No. 7, (July) 1950, pp. 259–63.

II

Techniques Applied

6

Effleurage

Effleurage is used more than any other of the massage techniques. It usually initiates each treatment. The evaluation which the physical therapist can make of the patient's soft-tissue with this technique can orient her better than a written or verbal report. During these initial strokes, sensitive fingers can explore for areas of tenderness and tightness. Effleurage is often interspersed between other strokes; it is used to progress from one area to another, and is the most common stroke used in concluding the treatment. It should therefore be mastered well, so that it can be performed with rhythm and confidence.

Description of effleurage
Any stroke which glides over the skin without attempting to move the deep muscle masses is called effleurage. The hand is molded to the part, stroking with firm and even pressure, usually upward.

Purpose of effleurage
This stroke is usually used for the beginning and ending of every massage as well as in-between all other strokes. It accustoms the patient to the touch of the physical therapist and allows sensitive fingers to search for areas of spasm and soreness. In given instances where extreme soreness is present it may be the only stroke employed. It serves to distribute evenly whatever lubricant is being used. Deep effleurage will also provide a passive stretch to given muscles or muscle groups.

Position of effleurage to the back

First see that the patient is comfortable, lying prone with the feet either off the end of the treatment table or supported at the ankle by a roll or pillow. A pillow under the abdomen is often a good idea and the arms may be placed wherever they are most comfortable. The head may be turned to either side.

In cases where it is difficult for a patient to lie down and get up, he can be treated in a sitting position. If this is done, he can rest his arms and head against the treatment table and they can be supported by pillows if necessary. Naturally, he must be seated on a stool or sideways on a chair so that the back can be free for treatment.

Draping for massage to the back

The patient is asked to loosen or remove any clothing which might interfere with the therapist's massage. This can be done after he has been covered with a sheet. If he needs assistance it should be given when he asks for it or if the physical therapist notices that he needs assistance. It is usually easier for the patient to loosen all clothing before turning to lie prone. The therapist then pulls the sheet down to the level of the coccyx, being careful not to expose the gluteal cleft. The sheet can be tucked over the edge of the patient's clothing or pajamas in order to protect them from the lubricant. This draping will suffice for these early practice techniques. If the low back is involved the entire gluteal area should be massaged. This is discussed more thoroughly in Part II, Chapter 12, pages 73–74.

Application of effleurage to the back

Since powder leaves a clear pattern to follow, apply it using enough so a pattern can be seen. Remember that too much powder will prevent good contact between the hand of the therapist and

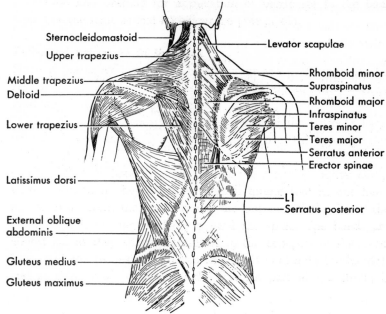

(From a sketch by Barbara Teasdale.)

Figure 1
Muscles of the back.

the skin of the patient. Place both hands on the patient's back at
the level of the coccyx, with the heel of the hand close to the spine
and the fingers pointing outward. Make sure the whole hand is
relaxed so that the entire palmar surface of the hand touches the
patient's body. Allow the hands to glide slowly along the erector
spinae group, being careful to avoid the spinous processes. As the
neck is approached, the hands move upward to the base of the skull.

The return stroke downward may have lighter pressure progressing laterally, with the fingers molding over and in front of the

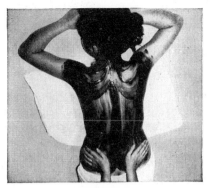

Figure 2
Fingerpaint pattern of effleurage.

shoulder to encompass the whole upper trapezius. As the stroke progresses, it follows the fibers of the upper trapezius to the shoulders and thence down the latissimus dorsi to the upper half of the gluteals.

Effleurage may be light or deep depending on the amount of pressure applied, but this pressure should be the same throughout the stroke, until the student learns more about how to vary it.

Points to check while practicing:

1. Is the patient *comfortable?*
2. Is the patient *relaxed?*
3. Are the *hands* of the *physical therapist* relaxed?
4. Is pressure even throughout each stroke?
5. Is the stance one of good body alignment, with weight over feet, or has the weight been allowed to fall forward over the treatment table?
6. Is *all* of the hand in contact with the patient?
7. Look at the powder patterns on the patient's back. Compare them with the illustrations above.

Variations of effleurage

Whenever the pressure on any effleurage stroke over any part of
the body is light, it is referred to as *light effleurage* regardless of
the part of the body to which it is applied or the pattern which
may be followed.

By the same token, any effleurage wherein the pressure is deep is
referred to as *deep effleurage.* Stroking and effleurage are terms
that may be used synonymously.

The student should attempt to make his pressure light throughout the entire stroke and again deep for the whole stroke. If he
can do this well he may then try to let his pressure start light
and increase until it is quite deep, tapering off again until it is
quite light at the end of the stroke. The student should then ask the
"patient" to guide him by telling him which pressure feels best, re-
membering that this "patient" is not one with an injured or arthritic
back, but an essentially healthy one.

Knuckling is a stroke particularly associated with the techniques
of Hoffa. In describing it he says:

> If the part to be treated is covered by thick fascia, effleurage is not
> deep enough. You need greater pressure, therefore the convex dorsal sides
> of the first interphalangeal joints must be used. Clench the fist in strong
> palmar flexion, the peripheral end of the knuckles should be upwards.
> Gradually bring the hand from plantar to dorsal flexion. Pressure is not
> continuous, but swells up and down, starting lightly and becoming
> stronger, then decreasing again in pressure. The hand must not adhere
> to the part but should glide over it lightly. Knuckling should only be used
> where there is enough room for the hand to be applied.*

Shingles refers to an alternate type of stroking in which one hand
follows the other with the strokes overlaying themselves one after
the other like the shingles on a roof. Thus, although contact with the

* Albert J. Hoffa: *Technik der Massage.* F. Enke, Stuttgart, 1900, p. 2.
Translation by Frances Tappan and Ruth Friedlander.

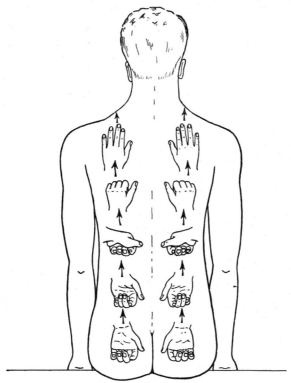

Figure 3
Knuckling.

patient is lost as each hand is lifted, the remaining hand maintains contact giving the patient a feeling of constant contact.

Bilateral tree stroking refers to both hands progressing simultaneously on either side of the back, from the spine laterally, and upward with short strokes that build like the branches growing from the trunk of a tree. (See right side of Frontispiece for fingerpaint pattern left by this stroke.)

Three-count stroking of the trapezius can be done with a rhythmical three-count stroke which begins at the origin of the lower trapezius, progressing with one hand toward the insertion. Simultaneously the other hand moves to the origin of the middle trapezius where it begins its stroke just as the other hand concludes, progressing toward the insertion of the middle trapezius. As soon as the first hand has completed its stroke of the lower trapezius, it pro-

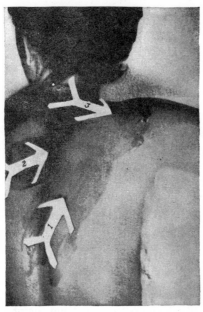

Figure 4
Three-count stroking
of the trapezius.

gresses *without contact* to the origin of the upper trapezius and strokes downward to the insertion to complete the third part of this three-count routine. This particular method of stroking the whole trapezius is rhythmical and relaxing when well done, but it must be timed like the shingles strokes so that, in spite of the lost contact, as each hand is raised, the patient feels constant contact because one hand is always stroking.

Horizontal stroking is particularly useful when applied to the low back. Place both hands lightly on the patient's back as shown in Figure 5. Using a stroke similar to effleurage, move the right hand forward and the left hand backward with firm pressure. When the hands have gone as far to the sides of the patient as possible, the stroke direction is reversed *without* changing the position of the hands. As the hands return to their original position a strong

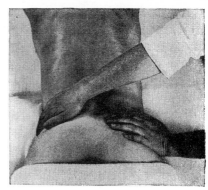

Figure 5
Horizontal stroking
to the low back.

lift and *push together* of the hips is executed. The returning hands continue all the way over to the opposite side of the patient, thus going from side to side across the back. No pressure should be placed over the spinous processes as the hands pass over them. Greatest pressure comes into the *lift* and *push together* of the low back as the hands pull upward and inward to meet and cross over the spinous processes and continue on down each side of the patient. This feels especially good to the patient who has a sacroiliac involvement.

Mennell's superficial stroking can be distinguished from light effleurage by its unidirectional flow "going either centripetally or centrifugally but never in both directions," and by its return stroke through the air which must be "controlled as for rhythm" taking as long as that part of the stroke which contacts the patient. Only the lightest possible pressure is used in this stroke (Mennell pp. 24–27).

Concluding stroke for relaxation is used if preparing the patient to relax for sleep. The treatment is concluded with long, light, effleurage strokes which start at the base of the skull, stroking directly over the spinous processes, going all the way down to the coccyx. Pressure must be very light but firm and the rhythm monotonous; too light pressure would stimulate rather than sedate. As one hand is about to complete the stroke near the coccyx, the other hand begins the next stroke starting at the base of the skull, giving the patient the feeling of continuous contact, with one hand beginning the next stroke before the other finishes. If this technique is kept up for a minute or two it helps the patient completely relax. The patient often obtains a tingling relaxation throughout the arms and legs which facilitates relaxation. Some patients will even fall asleep before the treatment is finished. If this technique is applied beyond two or three minutes it would tend to stimulate rather than relax so it should never be continued for long.

Summary

The effleurage strokes most often used in America today have been discussed. They should not limit the creative therapist who wishes to develop other types of effleurage strokes to suit the individual needs of the patient and to adjust the strokes described here on the back to all other parts of the body. The study of petrissage will teach the student how to combine these two massage techniques. While learning petrissage, effleurage should be interspersed between petrissage strokes for two reasons; to provide practice for the student, and to prevent "over petrissage" on any part of the body.

7

Petrissage

Petrissage is difficult to describe, but not difficult to perform. Contrary to effleurage which glides over the skin, petrissage strokes attempt to lift the muscle-mass and wring or squeeze it gently. Care should be taken not to work in one area too long before progressing to the next and not to pinch or bruise the tissues. It is easy for the beginner to forget these things and often, in a class of beginners, many black and blue spots appear. Students can help each other to adjust depth of pressure by reporting if real discomfort is felt. These strokes should be practiced on the back until they can be done rhythmically and with good close contact before being attempted on other parts of the body.

Description of petrissage

Petrissage consists of kneading manipulations which press and roll the muscles under the hands. It can be done with one hand, where the area to be kneaded is small, or it can be done with two hands on larger areas. It can even be done with two fingers on very small areas. There is no gliding over the skin except between progressions from one area to another.

Purpose of petrissage

This kneading motion of petrissage serves to "milk" the muscle of waste products which collect due to abnormal inactivity. It assists the venous return and in given instances it will also help to free adhesions.

Position and draping for application of petrissage to the back would be the same as that for effleurage (see p. 43).

Two-hand petrissage to the back

Since all petrissage is preceded by effleurage as a preliminary stroke, review the effleurage strokes, first stroking lightly and then working gradually into a deep effleurage.

Now place both hands firmly on one side of the patient's back, with the lower hand ready to start its motion over the upper portion of the gluteals.

Although each hand is going to describe a circle, counter-clockwise in direction, they do so with such timing that as one hand moves away from the spine across the muscles of the back, the other hand is moving medially toward the spine. The hands are almost *flat* as they shape themselves to the contours of the back. They pick the tissues up *between* the hands (not *with* the hands), and as they "pass" each other the forceful part of the stroke is

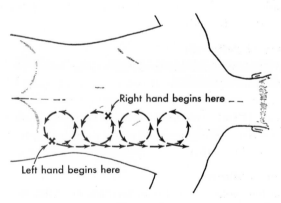

Figure 6
Petrissage of the back.

executed as the muscles are pressed downward against the ribs and rolled between the hands.

After about three repetitions of this stroke in one position, progress upward by allowing the lower hand to slide up to where the top hand has just been working, as the top hand glides upward to a new position.

Petrissage does not require much lubricant. The hands should cling to the part being massaged, picking up and pressing, sliding only when progressing, and even then with enough pressure so that fluids in the tissues are carried along with the stroke.

Variations of Petrissage

Alternating two-hand petrissage to the back

This type of petrissage for the back is very useful for following the direction of muscle fibers such as the trapezius.

Alternately use the index and middle fingers of one hand working with the thumb of the other hand. The thumbs are placed one above the other (see Fig. 7) and remain in this position, although

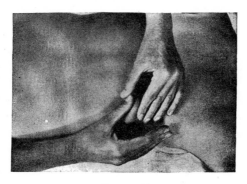

Figure 7
Alternating two-hand petrissage to the back.

the emphasis of each stroke is carried first by one hand and then the other. The fingers of one hand reach proximally, pick up the muscle, and move toward the opposite thumb. At the same time the thumb is pressing toward the proximal aspect of the muscle, moving toward the fingers. The opposite hand then repeats this same motion, and both hands alternately work from distal to proximal aspects of the muscle group (Barnett).

Two-finger petrissage on broad flat areas

Following the erector spinae muscle group up the back, grasp a small part between the thumb and first finger. Press it out as is done in other petrissage strokes. Although the movement is small, the whole motion should come through a relaxed arm.

Other variations of petrissage are best practiced on areas smaller to grasp. Positioning and draping are described on pp. 78–79 with the discussion of massage to the upper extremity. For purposes of this early practice they can be referred to briefly.

When applying any of the following techniques to areas of the body other than the back, "C" and "V" positions of the hand are used.

The C and V position names are derived from the C-like formation of the hand position as it grasps the arm or leg with the thumb in abduction and slightly flexed with the fingers cupped to fit the part being massaged. Pressure is exerted on the palm and the palmar surface of all fingers according to the contour of the part (Figs. 8–9). The wide or open C would be applied to the hand position where a large area such as the thigh is involved (Figs. 8, 32). The narrow, or closed C (Figs. 9–10) refers to the use of the same position when it is applied to an arm or smaller area. On very narrow areas the position is so narrowed that the thumb comes into adduction and the position is then referred to as the V position (Fig. 11).

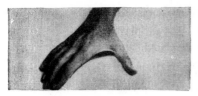

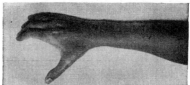

Figure 8
Open "C" position.

Figure 9
Closed "C" position.

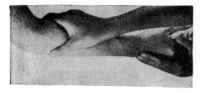

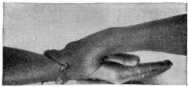

Figure 10
Closed "C" position.

Figure 11
"V" position.

One-hand petrissage

For use on smaller limbs (arms and children's legs) one hand is sufficient for petrissage. Place the hand *around* the part, picking up the muscle mass, using the *whole* hand. Lift the muscle away from the bone, squeezing gently upward and making small circular motions. Let the hand relax on the downward part of this small circle.

As with the two-hand petrissage, the rhythm should be slow and regular. Progression upward to a new position should follow three or four strokes. As the hand progresses, pressure is upward, carrying the venous return and lymph with it.

Since the biceps offers a distinctive, easily-grasped muscle, apply one-hand petrissage to the upper arm. Let the muscle belly fit into the palm of the hand while the thumb and fingers apply pressure to the upward part of the stroke.

Alternate one-hand petrissage

Another approach to petrissage of the upper arm may be accomplished by grasping the biceps in one hand and the triceps in the other. Using an alternate pattern of squeezing, petrissage both the flexors and the extensors with a soothing rhythm. As the one hand is relaxed the other is putting on pressure with the same, upward, circular strokes.

In circumstances where a certain amount of stimulation is indicated, this stroke can be used to advantage, progressing rather rapidly with each stroke working always in the direction of the venous flow.

Summary

Other variations of petrissage are included in Part III and will not be included here. These fine differences should not be attempted until the basic approach has been mastered. Later, if a student can do one technique better than the other, he can then be selective in the technique he prefers. While learning friction, both effleurage and petrissage should be interspersed, since students practicing on each other often work too deeply and bruise the tissues.

8

Friction

Although massage could consist of only effleurage and petrissage, friction is necessary if the therapist wants to reach beneath the more superficial tissues. Storms and Cyriax feel that friction is the most important massage technique and base most of their massage treatment around this stroke. When used correctly it permits the therapist to work into the deeper tissues gradually, judging by the patient's reaction how far to go.

Description of friction
Friction is performed by small circular movements with the tips of the fingers, the thumb, or the heel of the hand, according to the area to be covered. Small flat ellipsoids are described which penetrate into the depth of the tissue, not by moving the fingers on the *skin* but by moving the tissues *under* the skin.

Purpose of friction
Friction is used to massage deep into the joint spaces or around bony prominences such as the patella. It is especially useful around a well-healed scar to break down adhesions between the skin and tissues which are beneath it. It *cannot* affect a deep fibrositis such as might form within a muscle belly.

Application of friction to the back
Arrange the patient as for a back massage and begin the treatment with effleurage and then petrissage.

Using the ball of each thumb, place one on each side of the spinous processes of the back. Any level of the back will do for a spot to learn the technique. Press as deeply as the patient can tolerate without pain, describing small circles with a force that comes down through the arm from the shoulder. These small circles do not slide across the skin (as effleurage does), nor do they "pick up" or "squeeze" (as petrissage does). They gradually press into the

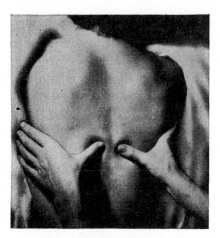

Figure 12
Friction.

tissues, becoming deeper as the patient develops tolerance to the pressure. Pressure should never be released suddenly.

Progress upward after about three cycles, following bilaterally upward to the side of the spinous processes, and in the muscular spaces between the transverse processes. The student learning friction should never practice too long in one spot because his attempts to obtain deep pressure may cause bruising until he learns his own strength and adjusts his technique.

Pressure follows up either side of the spine, avoiding the bony prominences. Following deep friction, effleurage stroking of the immediate area may be done with the thumbs to help the patient relax.

While the thumbs are doing the major portion of the work with this technique, the rest of the hand rests lightly on the back. It does not brace the thumb.

Variations of Friction

Cross fiber manipulation
Deep friction-like strokes which apply pressure *across* the muscle fiber, rather than along the longitudinal axis of the muscle fibers, can be applied to the erector spinae group of the back. Unlike typical friction strokes the thumb moves across the skin with deep short strokes.

Place one thumb close to the spinous process and stroke outward with deep pressure. Follow this stroke immediately by doing likewise with the other thumb, working thus, alternately up the back.

This type of manipulation can be done over any localized area, particularly in the presence of nodules or localized tightness.

Storms' technique
Harold D. Storms of Toronto, Canada, has developed a stroke which he used both for diagnostic and therapeutic measures, particularly for fibrositic nodules.

The cushions of the finger tips or the ball of the thumb do not slide over the skin, instead they hold position on the skin, the short stroke being made possible by moving the connective tissue *under* the skin.

This stroke varies from the previously described friction strokes in that the direction of the stroke is always parallel to the muscle fibers, rather than circular or cross-fiber in direction. Storms specifies also that as soon as the spasm *begins* to soften, massage should stop for that day.

Cyriax's friction for fibrositic muscles

Cyriax recommends deep friction given to the site of the lesion, which may or may not be within the painful area outlined by the patient.

There are four ways in which the therapist may use her hand to provide friction *across* the fibers of the structure being treated. Muscle, ligament, and joint capsule require friction administered perpendicularly to the long axis of the fibers composing them. The thicker and stronger the tissue the greater the exactitude needed.

This can be done using the index finger crossed over the middle finger; using the finger tips of the middle and ring fingers; using opposed fingers and thumb in a pinching position; or by using the superimposed thumbs, with the one thumb reinforcing the other.

Summary

Although there may be times when friction is not used at all in giving massage, there are other times when effleurage and petrissage merely prepare the tissues for the deeper application of friction. If the therapist will concentrate on working into this depth *gradually* the patient will be able to tolerate more depth. By the same token when the therapist is "letting go" it should be gradual and slow so that the patient experiences no sudden change. The following discussion of tapotement will further develop the students knowledge of massage technique. As stated previously, all techniques learned thus far should be interspersed in practice of tapotement since, until the student has mastered the art of "bouncing off," the patient may take a slight "beating."

9

Tapotement

Although tapotement is not used as often as the other masage techniques, it does have its place and requires practice to be able to perform it well.

Because of the indiscriminate use of tapotement in beauty salons and as often shown in motion pictures on prizefighters, and because of the unscientific claims that excess flesh can be "beaten off," many therapists shun using it at all. It should not, because of this, be ignored. If anything, emphasis on doing it correctly, and definition of its proper use, should be stressed.

Description of tapotement
Any series of brisk blows, following each other in a rapid, alternating fashion, come under the broad term of tapotement. Included under this heading are hacking, cupping, slapping; beating, tapping, and pincement.

Purpose of tapotement
Tapotement is used when stimulation is desired. Since most therapeutic massage is for purposes of relaxation, tapotement is often not a part of the general routine of massage. In athletics where stimulation is usually the purpose of massage it plays a more important role. Occasionally the apathetic patient may receive slight stimulation and a pleasant sensation of well-being following massage which has been terminated with tapotement.

Application of Tapotement to the Back

Hacking

Before reading the following instructions, shake the hands, letting the wrist, hand, and fingers relax and "flip up and down." No attempt should be made to hold the fingers together or the hands or wrist in any particular position. If relaxation is complete, it will be noticed that the hands fall into a neutral plane of motion which neither supinates nor pronates the forearm.

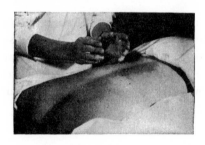

Figure 13
Starting position.

When relaxation is complete, an alternate direction of each arm can be started, the one moving up while the other moves down, still keeping the hands relaxed and shaking them.

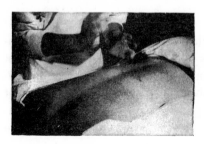

Figure 14
In motion.

Approach the patient now, holding the hands so that the palms are parallel, striking the back with a series of soft, but brisk blows, using the backs of the third, fourth, and fifth finger tips. Use both hands, alternating them and striking rapidly. Done correctly the effect is one of *pleasant* stinging and stimulation.

Figure 15
On contact.

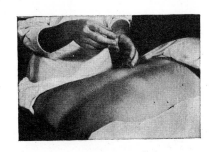

Progress from the hips upward to the shoulder and then back downward to the hips again. Tapotement should never be done over the kidneys. For increased stimulation effect, use alcohol applied with one or two rapid, light effleurage strokes just previous to the hacking strokes.

Cupping
This stroke is applied with the same rhythmical, rapidly alternating force, changing only the position of the hands to apply the blow with a cupped hand. Cup the hand so that thumb and fingers are slightly flexed, and the palmar surface contracted. Strike the back with the palm of the hand. This presumably causes a slight vacuum with each blow and some people believe it may loosen the broad flat areas of scar tissue. It makes a rather loud noise if done correctly, which could be detrimental or useful, depending on the psychological situation at hand.

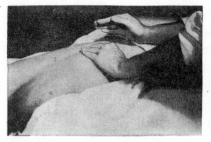

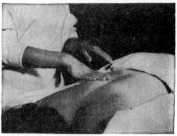

Figure 16
Cupping.

Figure 17
Slapping.

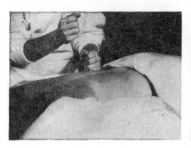

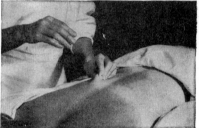

Figure 18
Beating.

Figure 19
Pincement.

Slapping

In the same manner, but using an open rather than a cupped hand,
strike gently but briskly with the fingers rather than the palm of the
hand.

Beating

The same stroke can be done using the hypothenar eminence of the
hand, with the fist closed. Care should be taken to keep the force of
the blows light and "bounding" in effect rather than jarring.

Pincement

Likewise, rapid, alternate, *gentle* pinching which picks up small portions of tissue between the thumb and first finger can be done.

Tapping

Tapping is done with the ends of the fingers, using sharp taps that make use of moderate fingernails, or padding the tap by using the pads of the fingers if the patient cannot tolerate the sharpness of the ends of the fingers.

10

Vibration

Vibration has been developed in Europe to the extent that European therapists can often execute this technique with a high degree of skill. Although it is described here for those who want to use it, it is the opinion of this author that vibration can be better given with an electrical vibrator, with the exception of the very gentle vibration mentioned in treating peripheral neuritis and poliomyelitis.

Description of vibration
A fine tremulous movement, made by the hand or fingers placed firmly against a part, will cause the part to vibrate.

Purpose of vibration
Vibration is often used for a soothing effect, particularly in treating peripheral neuritis. The treatment follows the path of the nerve. Vibration for this purpose must be very gentle and rhythmical, using fine vibrations. It has been used in Europe for poliomyelitis patients with such delicacy that the vibrating hand does not even touch the part, but merely flutters above it.

Application of vibration to the back
Use the same draping and position previously described. Place one hand anywhere on the back with the finger tips slightly apart. The rhythmical, trembling movement comes from the whole forearm, through the elbow, but the wrist and finger joints are kept stiff. The elbow should be slightly flexed. This vibrating motion should

be more up and down, than side to side. Heavy pressure should be avoided, especially if used with peripheral neuritis patients.

Variations of Vibration

When following the path of a nerve for a soothing effect, an effleurage type of stroke done with just the finger tips is employed, adding the vibration to the light effleurage stroke. Pressure can even be made so light that there is almost no contact of the hand with the part, and the vibrating hand moves almost out of contact. With extremely hypersensitive cases this technique has been credited with bringing a soothing effect.

Shaking

Another variation of vibration in a much coarser degree is useful for patients who have difficulty relaxing. It often helps to pick up the muscle belly (especially the biceps or gastrocnemius) and gently shake it back and forth. It is also helpful at times to shake the entire limb gently in order to encourage relaxation.

Summary

Vibration should not be used at all if the therapist has not put the time and effort into learning to do it well. Done well it can be extremely soothing, but poorly done it will only cause frustration and impatience on the part of both patient and therapist. It is difficult to learn well, and seldom used in America. Emphasis given to this technique must be decided by the therapist.

This concludes the basic strokes of massage. The following chapters describe how these techniques can be applied to any part of the body for therapeutic effects.

II

General Procedures of Massage

When all of the strokes in the preceding chapter have been learned, there must be practice in applying them to all parts of the body. The individual differences of each patient and each condition treated necessitates constant adjustment of the treatment. This may vary from day to day, therefore no set routine can be followed.

Begin cautiously

Generally massage begins with light effleurage which follows the venous flow. Do not massage directly over the most tender areas or the actual site of injury, but proximal to it. As the patient grows accustomed to the touch of the therapist the involved area can then be cautiously approached. When the patient can tolerate rather deep effleurage the therapist may work into petrissage. This may be light or deep depending again on the extent of the involvement and tolerance of the patient.

If other techniques such as friction, cross-fiber manipulation, and tapotement are used, they follow the use of effleurage and petrissage. Effleurage is usually interspersed with other strokes and is the stroke ordinarily used to begin and finish a massage treatment.

In concluding the treatment, strokes which work gradually from deep to light should be used. Tapotement, if used at all, is most often given at the end of the massage treatment as a terminal touch. It is not usually used in therapeutic situations unless on stump ends. It is often used in athletic situations or for other stimulating purposes.

68

Use originality

The therapist must use his own judgment and originality to find the correct approach to be used with each patient. In many cases that which "feels good" will be a strong factor in choice of strokes. At other times whether it "feels good" or not, certain techniques will be necessary. Each stroke has a purpose. It becomes the responsibility of the therapist to judge from the tissues beneath the working hands which techniques to select; how deep the pressure should be; how gentle the stretching must be; when to progress from one stroke to another; and when to progress from one area to another.

It is never wise to spend too long in one small area. It is more advisable to massage the whole general area, coming back to the areas of tenderness often.

Know the objectives

The objective of each treatment should be kept in mind. Each case will have one or more problems, such as pain, limited motion, swelling, etc., which require special attention.

If massage is given for a sedative purpose, the strokes will be slow and rhythmical, using effleurage and petrissage with pressure that is not too deep. Slow, rhythmical effleurage with the part in elevation will reduce edema. If the desired effect is stimulation, speed of the stroke can be increased and deeper pressure can be used.

Follow muscle groups

The therapist needs to be aware of the muscle groups involved in each case. The usual procedure is to massage each muscle group (for example the flexors of a joint), applying effleurage and petrissage which can be followed by friction or any other special strokes which may seem indicated. Each muscle group should be "stroked off" with effleurage before proceeding to the next muscle group.

There are times when the therapist may need to approach the involved part by some division other than by muscle groups but this should only be an exception to the rule. The therapist may massage the anterior aspect of the body before approaching the posterior, in order to avoid asking the patient to turn over more than once. In so doing, the therapist should still be aware of the muscle or muscle group that is being massaged.

When muscular tightness is present, friction to the tendons, toward their insertion, will help relieve protective muscle splinting against pain.

Summary

Aside from these general remarks, it is not the feeling of this author that specific instructions can be given for any specific involvement (as Cyriax does). The therapist must be aware of the basic conditions that exist, such as pain, swelling, limited motion, etc., and treat these symptoms, regardless of whether they are caused by surgery, accident, or illness. After learning to apply massage techniques to the various areas of the body, the student will then be ready to study the cases in Chapter 13. He will begin to learn how to plan individual routines for specific situations.

12

Massage Applied to Specific
Areas of the Body

As emphasized in the previous chapter, each patient will display different symptoms even though the diagnosis may be the same. These suggestions, pertaining to each of the different areas of the body, merely point out some specialized approaches that make it easier for the therapist to apply the techniques. Trained, sensitive fingers searching for muscle spasm, nodules, tightness, and painful areas will be able to locate the individual symptoms of each patient.

Massage of the Back

Using the positions and draping described on page 43, effleurage and petrissage to the following muscles or muscle groups should be given:

Erector spinae	Trapezius
Latissimus dorsi	Rhomboids
Gluteals	Levator scapuli

Light effleurage to all of the above will orient the therapist to tense or painful areas to be given more detailed consideration later in the treatment. All strokes should follow the muscle fibers. Any or all of the techniques learned previously can be applied. A variety of strokes and patterns can be selected to treat the individual complications that each patient may have.

71

Massage of the Low Back

Position

When positioning the patient for a low back involvement the therapist should consider putting the spine in slight flexion by placing a pillow under the abdomen with the patient face-lying. Some patients cannot lie comfortably in this position. If moving is difficult or impossible the therapist must adapt the techniques so that the patient can be treated side-lying or even lying flat on his back. Therefore effleurage and petrissage should be practiced with the patient lying in all positions. This involves applying the strokes at different angles. The therapist may find the height at which he has been working needs to be adjusted by stepping on or off a low platform.

When lying on his side, the patient should have the top leg well supported. The top arm should be supported in a position where the therapist is sure he is not using it to help maintain the side-lying position. Pillows under the leg and arm will not only give them support, but also will keep the patient from falling forward when pressure is applied to the back.

Draping

Draping is no different in principle for any of these positions. A sheet or towel should keep any part which is not being treated covered as neatly as possible.

Application of technique

Because of heavy fascia in the low back area, many patients can tolerate rather heavy pressure. The piriformis is often in spasm and only deep friction through relaxed gluteals can exert any pressure on it. The amount of direct mechanical effect on this muscle is debatable.

Massage of the Glutei

Many people will be sensitive to massage of the glutei, therefore some special approaches should be discussed.

Draping

As little of the area should be exposed as possible. Only that which is necessary should be left uncovered. The therapist can often work under the sheet. If only one side is involved a sheet can be placed so it covers the entire other half of the body, including the gluteal cleft.

Application of technique

The therapist can help the patient adjust to the touch of her hands by working on either the lower extremity or the back, stroking gradually toward the gluteal area. This is contrary to the usual approach of massaging the proximal area first. The purpose of reversing this procedure is to help the patient adjust to treatment of this area.

Strokes to this area need to be heavy due to the large muscle-mass. They should follow the direction of the muscle fibers for each of the gluteal muscles. Follow the usual sequence of effleurage, petrissage, and friction where indicated. Deep effleurage strokes which go around the acetabulum and the tuberosity of the ischium should be included. It is difficult to reach through this large muscle-mass to palpate the piriformis which is often in spasm, but with relaxation of the gluteals it can sometimes be accomplished.

Friction can often be tolerated about the lumbosacral and sacro-iliac regions but should be done carefully since these areas are often sensitive. Friction should also be done over the area of the greater sciatic notch, the ischial tuberosities, and the area between the iliac crest and the greater trochanter and around the greater trochanter.

If the patient must lie on his back the problem for the therapist is to reverse her technique from applying pressure downward to that of reaching under the patient and applying pressure upward. Effleurage is fairly easy to do in this fashion but petrissage is much more difficult. One hand can effect the circular motion of the usual two-hand petrissage, progressing up the back. Friction is also easy to apply, using the tips of the fingers with the palm facing the patient, working with the typical small circles of friction or with a cross-fiber technique.

Practice of massage to the back should be done with the patient in all positions, even seated with the head resting against the treatment table with a pillow on it, because patients with back involvement often find lying down very difficult.

Massage of the Cervical and Thoracic Spine

Position

Patients requiring massage of the thoracic or cervical spine are often more comfortable lying face down, with a pillow under the chest, and with the head supported by a small, rolled towel in a neutral position. Patients have a difficult time getting comfortable if they have pain in this area. The therapist often discovers that the patient can find a comfortable position better by himself than by being told in which position to lie. If it is impossible to find a comfortable position lying down, the massage can be given with the patient in a sitting position, leaning on a pillow placed on the treatment table. Either position is acceptable. Possibly the sitting position is a little more convenient for the therapist. The arms may be placed wherever comfortable as long as they do not support the weight of the patient and are relaxed. In some instances the head may be supported with a Sayre head sling for support or slight stretching combined with massage. Some patients will be more comfortable in a back-lying position with the therapist standing at the head of the treatment table.

Draping

There should be no clothing on the upper back. Women may be given a hospital gown which splits down the back but protects the rest of the body if treated in a sitting position. If the patient is lying down, the draping is the same as it has been for the other techniques applied to the back.

Application of technique

All of the variations of effleurage described previously can be applied to this area. The three-count stroking of the upper trapezius (p. 48) is especially useful. Stretching can be applied to the upper trapezius. Use one hand to stabilize the head and the other to give a deep effleurage stroke which goes from the origin to the insertion of the upper trapezius. Pressure should be deep enough to stretch the muscle fibers but never deep enough to cause pain. Care should be taken that the stabilizing hand does not push the head away. It maintains good alignment of the cervical spine, serving to hold the head still so that the stretch is accomplished by pushing the shoulder downward and not by pushing the head away.

Sayre head sling and stretching

In cases where the Sayre head sling has been prescribed, effleurage strokes for the upper trapezius can be applied while the patient is receiving traction from the head sling.

Care should be taken to see that pressure is so placed that normal alignment of the cervical spine is not displaced.

Verbal instructions for relaxation will assist the patient in getting maximal benefit from this type of treatment.

All petrissage techniques can be adapted to this situation, even the one-hand petrissage which can be used on the upper trapezius. Two-hand petrissage can also be done on the muscle-mass of the upper trapezius which can be grasped with the hands molding over the anterior aspects of the muscle. If deep petrissage is done with upward progression toward the head, it should be followed by deep effleurage strokes downward to assure good venous return. The therapist should watch the complexion of the patient, and if the face is flushed, only downward pressure should be used.

Friction may be used as previously described (pp. 57–59), following up the spine on either side of the spinous processes all the way up to the occiput. Any involvement of the upper back or neck is apt to cause marked tenderness at the occipital protuberance. Friction therefore is cautiously applied around the tendinous insertion, or not done at all if the patient cannot tolerate this type of pressure.

Mennell refers to "sensitive deposits" which can be felt under the exploring hand of the therapist (Mennell, p. 474). These deposits are often found in the muscle bellies in this area and can be treated as described by Mennell or Storms. Storms' methods have already been discussed (pp. 59–60). Mennell advocates the use of frictions which begin gently at the periphery of the sensitive area and gradually approach the center of it. This should be followed by deep petrissage. Cross-fiber manipulation may also be used in a similar fashion.

Although *tapotement* and *vibration* may be used, these strokes are not routinely part of treatment.

Massage of the Chest

Position
The patient should be back-lying with due consideration for the relaxation of all muscles that originate or insert from the chest. Slight flexion at the knees would tend to relax the abdominals. Pillows under the arms will relax the pectorals. A pillow under the head should relax the muscles of the neck.

Draping
A towel or sheet should cover the side not being treated.

Application of techniques

Any or all of the techniques described except tapotement, may be applied to the chest. Because of the many types of surgery or injury that could be treated in this area, no particular approach to special muscle groups can be outlined. Involved muscles should be treated by groups. Scar tissue, especially following mastectomy, may often be the major concern. Stretching techniques should be applied if the shoulder has been held in protective splinting leading to tightness. In this event consideration should be given to those posterior muscles which may also be tight.

Massage of the Abdomen

Position

The patient should be back-lying with the knees in slight flexion and supported so that the hip flexors and abdominal muscles are relaxed. The head may be resting on a pillow.

Draping

A towel or sheet should cover the upper part of the patient, and another one the lower part of the patient so that only the abdomen is exposed.

Application of technique

Orders are almost never received for abdominal massage. There was a time when it was ordered for constipation. This author does not recommend it, but includes it for those who might want instruction.

Gentle effleurage strokes should be used to accustom the patient to the touch of the therapist. All strokes should follow the direction of the colon, as it ascends on the right, crosses, and then decends on the left. Gradually increase pressure (but never too heavily). Light petrissage may follow the same pattern followed again by effleurage.

It is usually easier for the therapist to stand on the patient's right side.

Friction, with precaution against going too deeply, can then follow. Use circular strokes which follow the direction of the colon. Complete the treatment with light effleurage in the same direction.

Caution: Abdominal massage could cause serious complications in the event of pregnancy or appendicitis. It is considered unwise therefore to practice abdominal massage on each other in classes of students studying massage.

Massage of the Upper Extremity

Position

Range of motion in the shoulder joint may be the deciding factor as to whether the patient will be treated in a sitting or lying position. If there is tightness of the pectorals, but not inhibiting pain, it is well to treat the patient sitting with the arm supported. This puts a slight stretch on the muscle while the patient is being treated. The amount of stretch can be increased by raising the height of the arm or lowering it if it cannot be tolerated. If severe pain, such as with bursitis, prevents this position, the arm may rest on a pillow in the patient's lap or on a lower table. These patients are often more comfortable lying down.

If the hand or wrist is involved, the hand is usually supported by a small roll or towel, so that it rests with the wrist slightly extended. The fingers, if relaxed, will rest in partial flexion. This position also puts the fingers slightly off the table, which protects the finger tips from bumping on the table if they are hypersensitive.

Draping

Only the arm being treated should be left uncovered. A towel or a sheet may be used to cover the patient in such fashion that it will not slip, especially if the patient is in a sitting position. If the entire arm is to be treated, the draping should cross the shoulder not being treated and be fastened securely with a safety pin. Sleeves of the patient should never be pushed up. The shirt or blouse should be taken off to prevent tight clothing from inhibiting the venous return.

Application of technique

The greatest change to be noticed in adapting the strokes to the arm and hand is in the position of the therapist's hand. As previously described (see page 54), the hand is open to cover the wide surfaces of the back. On the arm and hand a closer position will be used to encompass the smaller area with close contact, using either the C or the V position (see page 54).

Upper arm

Muscles or muscle groups to be considered in massage of the upper arm would include those of the cervical and upper back if the shoulder were involved. (See p. 69 for general procedures.) These muscles are often tense from muscle splinting to avoid pain in the injured or involved aim. If so they should also be treated. Muscles of the arm would include the pectorals, serratus, deltoid, triceps, and biceps. In addition to massage for each muscle or muscle group, the joints should be considered. Care should be taken not to place deep pressure into the joint or over bony prominences.

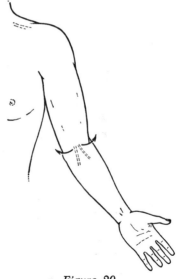

Figure 20

In addition to those techniques already described, Dicke's stretching of the elbow joint provides mild, passive stretching of the pronator teres and the brachioradialis (Figure 20). Bimanual stretching of the elbow joint can be done with the patient's elbow slightly flexed. The therapist holds the olecranon and pronator teres in one hand, and the brachioradialis in the other. The pull outward is accomplished as the therapist's fingers flex, stretching these two tendons simultaneously (Dicke, p. 28).*

Lower arm

In the lower arm the flexors of the wrist and fingers can be treated as a group. The extensors comprise the other major muscle group to be treated. Those muscles which cross both the elbow and the wrist should be considered. Both of these joints should be included in the massage and any limited range of motion should be *gently* stretched using effleurage strokes which encourage increased range of motion.

If some of the muscles of the upper arm, such as the biceps, are involved due to muscle splinting or casting positions, the massage should include treatment of them also.

Hand

A common problem of the student therapist is the *overstretching* of the capsule in the small joints of the fingers. The fingers need to be stretched *gently*. A gentle, steady pull, combined with slow effleurage wherein the therapist's first finger surrounds most of the finger, while the thumb covers the dorsal aspect, will both feel good and be beneficial to the patient. However the "popping" of the joints can be very harmful and should be avoided. A Mennell type of passive motion, which gently encourages active motion and increases the range of motion can be combined with massage of the fingers. *Little good can come from overstretching.* It tears the tissues and causes increased swelling and pain.

The fingers are so small that massage is difficult. It must be practiced until it can be done well, for hand injuries are common and the swelling and limited motion that accompanies such injuries need treatment.

* These techniques and illustrations are adapted from the techniques of Elisabeth Dicke. Page numbers refer to her book, *Bindegewebsmassage.*

All strokes previously described can be adapted to these smaller areas and must be mastered.

Elisabeth Dicke's strokes so completely cover all aspects of massage to the hand that they are included here. However, she would never give the treatment described here without building up to it through massage of the back by her own specific methods, which are not discussed in this text (Dicke, p. 29). Most of these strokes would be applied by the soft pads of the therapist's finger tips.

In the event of swelling of the hand, any of these strokes which go against the venous flow should be done in reverse. This is the recommendation of this author and not described by Dicke. Dicke also recommends that these strokes be done a specific number of times each. This author would rather leave this to the judgment of the therapist.

Position
The patient's hand should rest comfortably in either pronation or supenation, depending on the involvement.

Application of technique
To perform these strokes the therapist uses the soft pad of the middle finger, pulling with some depth, from proximal to distal. Both thumbs of the physical therapist rest on the patient's wrist with no pressure during these strokes.

As illustrated in Figure 21a, the first stroke pulls over the lower third of the flexor carpi radialis. The second stroke pulls over the palmaris longus (Fig. 21b). The third stroke pulls over the flexor carpi ulnaris (Fig. 21c).

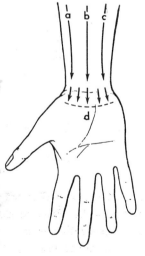

Figure 21

These are followed by short strokes over the volar ligament. Be careful not to press too deeply over the median nerve. Stabilize above the wrist. Get the pull by flexing the fingers. Start on the radial side and work toward the ulnar side (Fig. 21d).

Next follow short strokes over the transverse ligament across the heel of the hand from thenar to hypothenar eminences (Fig. 22a). Then long strokes are done over the palmar fascia, working deep to the interossei, pulling toward the fingers (Fig. 22b). Thenar strokes which are half ellipsoid are then given over the inner surface of the thenar eminence (Fig. 22c).

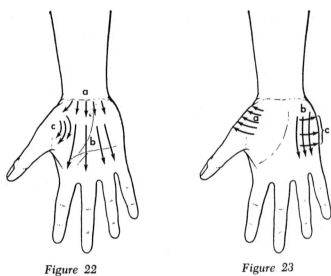

Figure 22   Figure 23

Transverse strokes are then done over the thenar eminence, working from the inner border outward toward the dorsal surface (Fig. 23a). Hypothenar strokes of a similar nature are done in a longitudinal direction (Fig. 23b) and in a transverse direction (Fig. 23c).

Small, interdigital, longitudinal strokes over the transverse palmaris ligament between the heads of the metacarpals should then be done (Fig. 24).

On the dorsum of the hand, short strokes should be done. The therapist anchors the thumb on the volar side starts radially over the ligamentum dorsalis and goes distally across the ligament adding gentle, passive extension of the wrist simultaneously (Fig. 25a).

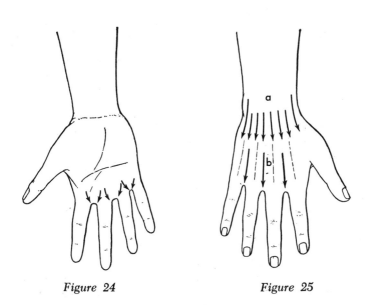

Figure 24   Figure 25

Next perform long, flat, gentle strokes over the interossei (Fig. 25b).

The following stroke is best done with the thumbs. It is a pull and counterpull to stretch the web between the fingers. One hand holds, while the other pulls the next finger away, providing gentle passive motion as well as stroking. Begin on the radial side and work toward the ulnar side. This should be done to both the volar and dorsal surfaces of the hand (Figs. 26 and 27).

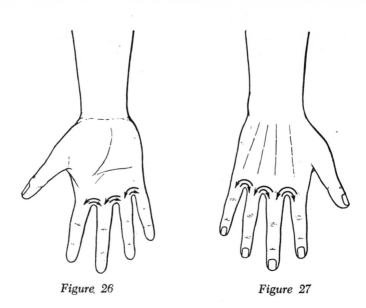

Figure 26   Figure 27

Massage of the fingers

Each finger should be massaged before going on to the next one.

Pull out the long tendons on the volar side of the fingers, stroking the tendon from metacarpophalangeal joint to the tip of the finger. Use one hand to support the patient's hand, to prevent hyperextension of the finger, and to get the proper pressure. *This pulling is not done by grasping the finger, but by stroking along the tendon* (Fig. 28a). Next perform small strokes on the medial and lateral borders of the first two phalanges (Fig. 28b). Follow this by stroking, proximal to distal, with a *little* stretch, over the collateral ligaments of each joint. *Do not pull* into the joint space or go beyond one joint at a time (Fig. 28c). Stretching of the small joints can be done (Fig. 28d).

Figure 29

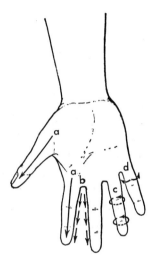

Figure 28

Stretch each joint of each finger by using both thumbs on the dorsal side and both third fingers, pulling outward (Fig. 29).

Next apply short strokes over the dorsal aponeurosis, beginning on the thumb. Stretch the long extensor tendons between each joint (Fig. 30). If the lumbercales are involved, stroke laterally between each joint.

Stretch the palmar fascia in the

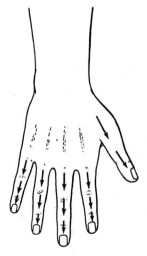

Figure 30

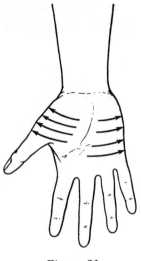

Figure 31

following fashion. With the thumbs on the dorsum of the patient's hand, the physical therapist pronates her own hands, stretching the palm or the patient's hand as the volar aspect of the patient's hand is supported by the hypothenar aspect of the therapist's hand. Start at the carpal area and work distally with each stroke (Fig. 31).

Although Dicke would not do so, this author recommends stroking off the entire extremity with effleurage, working from firm pressure gradually toward lighter pressure, and finishing with light effleurage strokes which follow the venous flow.

Massage of the Lower Extremity

Position

The patient receiving massage to the lower extremity should be lying down with the leg in neutral position or elevated in the event of swelling. There should be support at the knee and at the ankle. The foot should never be allowed to drop into plantar flexion, even though it is not necessarily involved. A pillow or drop-foot board should support the foot at about ninety degrees of dorsiflexion.

The patient may be face-lying if most of the treatment pertains to the posterior aspect of the leg. In this case the feet should be off the end of the treatment table and the lower leg supported so that the knee is in slight flexion, unless stretching of the hamstrings or gastrocnemii is indicated.

Draping

With an injured lower extremity it is often difficult for the patient to get out of pajamas or trousers. This can easily be handled by asking the patient to loosen the top and then advise him to hang onto the top of the sheet. Standing at the foot of the bed the therapist can then simply reach under the sheet and pull the trousers off. Always check to be sure the patient has a tight hold on the sheet or both the sheet and trousers will come when the trousers are pulled.

Occasionally there is demand for what is jokingly called "diaper" draping (Fig. 32). This can tactfully be managed by handing the patient a towel and asking him to place it so that it goes between the legs, covering him, both front and back. He can do this while protected by the sheet, working under it, or the therapist can leave the room while the patient drapes himself.

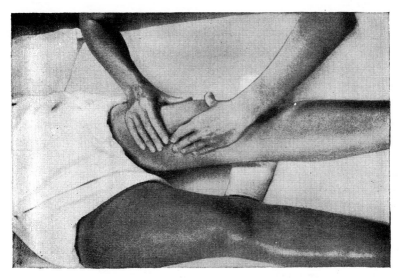

Figure 32
"Diaper" draping. Massage to the upper leg.

Application of technique

Mold the hands to the contours of the leg in applying effleurage and petrissage to the muscle groups involved. Care should be taken not to carry any strokes too high on the medial thigh. All of the principles mentioned in massage of the upper extremity also apply to the lower extremity (pages 78–79).

Upper leg

Muscle groups which should be considered in massage of the upper leg would include the gluteals if the hip is involved. The hamstrings, adductors, abductors, and quadriceps (Fig. 32) should be treated as groups and are usually involved in injuries to the hip or knee, or fractures of the thigh. The hip flexors are seldom massaged, but in the event of hip-flexion contractures they would benefit from treatment.

In addition to the techniques already described the following gentle stretching of the hamstrings and gastrocnemius, as done by Dicke, is a helpful technique (Dicke, p. 31).

Using both hands just above the popliteal space, lightly hold the tendons of the hamstrings with the finger tips. Lift and supinate both hands, gently stretching the tendons. This same technique can also be used for the two heads of the gastrocnemius, just below the popliteal space, but never working deep into the popliteal area.

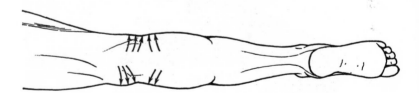

Figure 33

With injuries to the leg, the patella often lacks normal mobility. Care should be taken in cases of arthritis not to work too deeply with friction around the patella. In many cases, however, the therapist can use one hand to stabilize the patient's leg, while using the other hand to perform short, deep friction-like strokes which try to hook under the border of the patella (Dicke, p. 30).

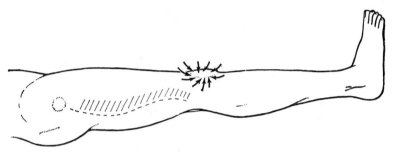

Figure 34

Pivot-like strokes, in which the heel of the hand acts as a pivot and the fingers stroke around the borders of the patella, can also be used (Dicke, p. 30).

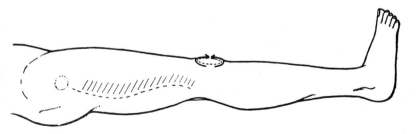

Figure 35

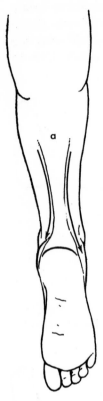

Figure 36

Lower leg

In the lower leg the tibialis anterior, tibialis posticus, the peroneals, and the gastrocnemius comprise most of the muscle masses to be treated as muscle groups. These muscle groups can be effleuraged, and petrissaged in preparation for detailed attention to be given any particular problems.

Elisabeth Dicke describes detailed strokes to cover the lower leg and foot (Dicke, p. 31). Those strokes which go against the venous flow should not, in the opinion of this author, be used if the foot is swollen, but could be applied in reverse. These strokes do, however, provide good gentle stretching to the tendons of the ankle.

Use bimanual stroking of the Achilles tendon, working from proximal to distal, beginning just distal to the belly of the muscle, pulling toward the back of the heel. The hands flex the foot slightly as they stroke (Fig. 36a).

Stroke the peroneus longus and brevis, around the malleolus, toward the dorsum of the foot. Stabilize the leg with the other hand.

In the same fashion, stroke the tibialis posticus and around the malleolus (Fig. 37a).

Complete the series by stroking bimanually both of these areas at the same time.

Foot

All of the principles brought out in the discussion of massage to the hand, particularly the special care taken when working with small joints (pp. 81–86), apply to massage of the foot.

Stabilize the foot with one hand. Use little strokes which go proximal to distal across the front of the ankle joint. Dorsiflex the ankle at the same time the stroke is done (Fig. 37b).

Apply short, little strokes between the metatarsophalangeal joints, going from proximal to distal, then medial to lateral (Fig. 37c).

If the toes are involved they will be done exactly as the fingers are done (see pp. 84–86).

Deep, little strokes should be done just in front of the heel, from the arch around the side of the foot, starting laterally and working medially. The same thing can be done going the other way, starting medially (Fig. 37d).

Short strokes can be done across the bottom of the heel.

Deep stroking of the plantar fascia can be done with long strokes

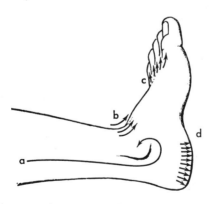

Figure 37

which cover the longitudinal arch from the heel up to the metatarso-phalangeal joint (Fig. 38a).

Plantar stroking may also go across the muscle fibers at right angles to the longitudinal arch (Fig. 38b).

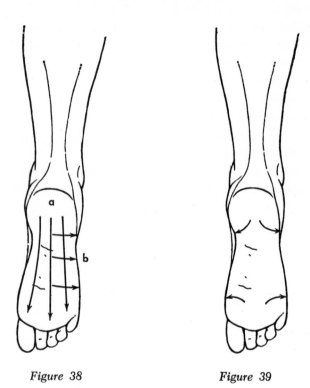

Figure 38   Figure 39

Bilaterally stretch both the top and bottom of the foot with a rolling motion of the hands; up and out on the proximal part of the foot. On the distal part of the foot, reverse direction to stretch the forefoot (metatarsal arch) in the opposite direction (Fig. 39).

Massage of the Face

Position

The patient may be lying down or seated, as preferred. The therapist stands behind the patient.

Draping

A small towel or hair net may be used to keep the hair away from the face during the treatment.

Application of technique

In cases of Bell's palsy the involved side of the face is often stretched, being pulled by the well muscles on the opposite side, especially around the mouth. In giving treatment, both sides should be massaged, since even the side of the face *not* paralyzed will have muscles which are tight. Support to lessen this pull should be given with the hand not being used to massage. This could alternate as both sides are treated.

Here again, Dicke's detailed instructions would be difficult to improve on (Dicke, pp. 32–33).

Bimanually stroke across the forehead, using three strokes from the hairline 'down to just above the eyebrows, moving from the center of the forehead toward the temple (Fig. 40a).

These same strokes can be done on only one side, while the other hand supports the opposite side.

Give a very soft pull from the lateral side of the eye into the hairline of the temple (Fig. 40b).

Anchor the heel of the hand on the cheek. Follow the upper eyebrow, stroking from medial to lateral toward the temple (Fig. 40c).

Repeat the same, following the lower rim of the eyebrow (Fig 40d).

Repeat a similar stroke just below the eye (Fig. 40e).

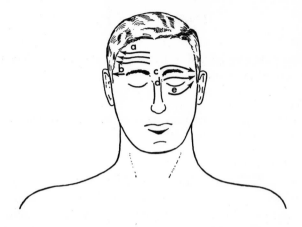

Figure 40

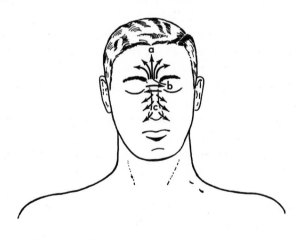

Figure 41

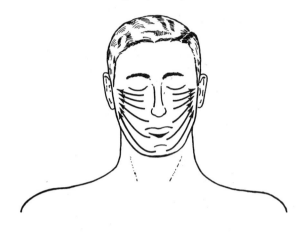

Figure 42

Give short little strokes upward between the eyes (Fig. 41a).

Pull from the involved side to the uninvolved side over the bridge of the nose. Reverse the direction also (Fig. 41b).

Bimanually stretch the nose, stroking from the center to each side. Work all the way down to the very tip of the nose (Fig. 41c).

Bimanually stroke the zygomaticus working from just under the eyes toward the mandible, stroking from front to back (Fig. 42).

In addition to these techniques of Dicke's, soft strokes directly over the closed eyes of the patient, pulling from the nose lightly over to the temple, can be very relaxing.

Petrissage can be done with two fingers in the smaller areas and with the thumb opposing the fingers over the fleshier parts of the face.

Gentle friction directly over the temples can be done.

Friction all around the hairline will release the tension caused by frowning or tightness of the muscles that originate or insert there.

With finger and thumb, the bridge of the nose can be stretched by pulling it outward.

Throughout all of these strokes, gentleness must be emphasized, and care taken not to put pressure directly over the eyes.

13

Cases for Analysis and Planning of Treatment Program

Regardless of the injury or illness of the patient, the therapist will be dealing with such conditions as pain, swelling, scar tissue, muscle spasm, fibrositic nodules, muscle splinting, poor skin condition following casting, contractures, and insufficiencies of circulation. Students of massage should be exposed to other courses such as pathology, orthopedics, surgery, and neurology, in order to understand the injuries and illnesses they will be dealing with. The following lists of indications and contraindications will give an overview of situations commonly treated by massage and those for which massage might do more harm than good.

Indications

Each indication should be considered with the view that there are times when it might *not* profit by massage. No therapist can be expected to do an adequate job of massage without a thorough understanding of the medical implications of each situation. If a certain effect is desired, the therapist must determine how it can be obtained.

In most of the following situations, massage would be indicated during a subacute phase *but not during an acute phase:*

Amputations
Arthritis
Burns
Bursitis

Myositis
Neurasthenia
Orthopedic and neurological
    situations

Contractures

Decubitus areas, and surrounding tissue

Facial paralysis (Bell's palsy)

Fractures

Insomnia

Long bed rest

Peripheral neuritis

Poliomyelitis

Postural deviations

Scar tissue (certain adhesions)

Strains and sprains

Tension headache

Torticolis

Contraindications

Massage should be used in the following conditions only under the most careful medical guidance, never by a new student unless most carefully supervised, and always with utmost caution.

Cardiac decompensation

Edema, obstructive or decompensated, also inflammatory or non-infectious

Hematomas

Herniated disc

Mental states, particularly depressive or manic

Nonunion fractures

Phlebitis

Postoperative

    tendon transplants

    orthopedic cases

    neurological cases

Severe lacerations

Spastic paralyses, such as: Parkinson's, multiple sclerosis, hemiplegias, paraplegias, congenital cerebral palsies, traumatic or post-surgical brain injuries, encephalitis

In many situations, the consequences of massage would be obvious to the therapist or student who understands its physiological or mechanical effects. The therapist must be aware of the damage which can be done by the indiscriminate use of massage.

Any of the conditions listed under indications which appear acute should be considered as contraindicated for massage. In addition to this the therapist should be sure that none of the following conditions exist before proceeding with massage:

Abdominal massage is contraindicated in the event of pregnancy, large hernias, or any possibility of peritonitis or appendicitis

Acute tubercular lesions, malignancies

Cellulitis

Certain neurotic conditions, especially emotional instabilities

Debilitating diseases

Edema due to heart decompensation or kidney ailments, synovitis, thrombus which may be dislodged, embolism, sinusitis

Fever

If it aggravates the patient's mental or physical condition

Localized acute infections

New surgery

Skin eruptions that may exacerbate

Undiagnosed friends without doctor's orders

Cases for Analysis and Planning of Treatment Program

The following cases include the diagnosis and treatment prescribed. They have been designed for the purpose of helping students of massage see the relationship between prescriptions and the planning that is needed to organize the massage treatment. By thinking these cases through for themselves, students will relate theory and practice. Greater confidence will be developed; professional attitudes will be strengthened; and effective reasoning and problem-solving ability will improve. The organization of a case will increase understanding of the disorder from which the patient is suffering.

Names, dates, record numbers, addresses, number and frequency of treatments, doctor's signatures, and dates for re-examination by the doctor have been deliberately ignored in the writing of the following cases. This is to focus attention on the massage. Such information is usually included in case reports, but here it would only be repetitive.

These cases include situations which involve many parts of the body and encompass conditions which are often treated by massage.

Users of this text who do not have adequate background or supplementary courses in anatomy, physiology and pathology, or are not taking a course with a qualified instructor who can competently guide and correct their plans, will profit little by this approach and should not attempt to analyze these cases by themselves. *In some instances these cases deliberately include situations which should not be massaged at all.* In these cases the student should be able to explain why massage would not be advisable. *In other cases inadequate or inaccurate information is provided.* In such cases the student should realize this and be able to state what questions would need to be answered before treatment could be given. *In several instances the treatment ordered is incorrect.* In these cases students should seek accurate treatment instructions, or be ready to recommend more appropriate treatment.

The following outline will assist students in the study of these cases. With the guidance and assistance of a qualified instructor, students will become more aware of the many things that have to be considered whenever they receive brief prescriptions. In each case the student should seek the following information:

1. Adequate description of the injury or illness
2. Significant dates of onset, surgery, casts, etc.
3. Necessary supportive measures: braces, crutches, and support needed during treatment
4. Treatment ordered (Is it adequate? Accurate?)
5. Precautions, indications and contraindications for the treatment ordered

In preparing themselves to massage these cases the students should consider:

1. Purposes of the treatment, such as reduction of swelling, increase in range of motion, reduction of pain, relaxation, etc.

2. Creation of relaxed environment, establishment of good patient-therapist relationship

3. Additional information that might be needed

4. Positioning and draping to be used

5. Assistance with dressing and undressing

6. Choice and use of lubricant

7. Organization of the massage treatment to include:
   a. Efficient use of time and equipment
   b. Area to be treated
   c. Direction, rhythm, and choice of strokes
   d. Pressure to be used, tolerance of patient to pressure
   e. Body mechanics of the therapist
   f. Termination of treatment, equipment to replace, cleaning up treatment table, arrangements for next appointment, etc.
   g. Other types of treatment given in addition to massage

8. Evaluation of effectiveness of treatment (What observations can be made that will indicate whether or not the objectives of treatment have been accomplished?)

The first case has been analyzed as a sample of the way these cases can be used:

Diagnosis

This three-year-old boy has received a severe burn to the right wrist. There is extensive scar tissue and flexion contractures at the wrist joint.

Treatment

Massage to the right forearm and hand, in preparation for stretching.

Description of injury

The description does not tell how the boy was burned nor when, nor how extensively the wrist is involved except that it was extensive enough to leave a scar and cause contractures at the wrist. Some of this could be found out quickly by examining the patient. Usually it is helpful to know how the accident happened. Such information could be obtained from the doctor or the patient's chart.

Significant dates

There is no indication of the date of the accident. This could probably be found by checking the patient's chart.

Support

No support should be needed other than for the comfort of the patient.

Treatment ordered

There is no order for heat preceding massage, nor is there an order to stretch. This should be cleared with the doctor and permission asked to combine stretching with massage. Permission should be sought to initiate an exercise program. It would seem that the finger flexors would also be tight. The therapist should seek permission to treat the whole situation.

Precautions

Be assured that the scar tissue is strong enough to permit this type of treatment and seek further information as to the extent of the deep scar tissue. Review the pathology of burns. (See W. A. D. Anderson: *Pathology*, 3rd ed., The C. V. Mosby Co., St. Louis, 1957. First, second and third degree burns, pages 133–34.)

Purpose of treatment

The purpose of massage in this case would be to promote relaxation, stretch tissue, encourage active motion, improve local blood supply, and increase range of motion.

Patient-therapist relationship
During the get-acquainted stage, gaining this little boy's confidence will be more important than the amount of range of motion gained. Care should be taken not to frighten him by causing undue pain. If he is afraid of white uniforms it might even be wise to wear street clothes until he is fully aware of what his treatment program involves.

Additional information needed
There is need to know the depth of the burn, how it happened, whether the elbow flexors are also tight, whether the finger flexors are involved, and the condition of the scar tissue.

Position
Since the patient is three years old he would probably be comfortable sitting on a treatment table with a pillow in his lap. This would put him high enough for the therapist to work with him easily. He might also be comfortable lying down on the treatment table, letting his arm rest on it.

Draping
Remove his shirt. Leave the undershirt on if it has no sleeves. Put a towel about the shoulders.

Assistance with dressing
Let the parents help him until he is acquainted with the therapist.

Lubricant
Use cocoa butter which is thought to be good for scar tissue.

Organization of treatment
   Time. Allow time to get acquainted for the first treatment; possibly thirty minutes, later massage could probably be done in about fifteen minutes.
   Area to be treated. If the elbow is also tight from protective positioning, the entire arm should be included in the massage. The upper

arm and elbow should be massaged before concentrated work on the wrist and hand is done.

Choice of strokes. Treatment of the upper extremity would be done as described on pages 78–86 of this text. In addition to this, deep effleurage strokes which stretch while they stroke should be carried out. By working into it gradually the patient will tolerate greater stretching. Stretching should never exceed the pain tolerance of the patient and should begin and end gradually. If there is no swelling, stretching strokes may pull downward against the venous flow. These should be followed by effleurage strokes which go with the venous flow. Keeping in mind that massage cannot break up deep adhesions or scar tissue, active motion (if permission was obtained for active exercise) should be encouraged. Much of the tightness present may be due to protective muscle splinting against pain. If this is so, good results can be expected. Treatment should be concluded by effleurage to the entire arm, working from deep pressure to light.

Pressure. Pressure should stay well within the tolerance of the patient.

Body mechanics of the therapist. Body mechanics of the therapist should be no problem with the patient on the treatment table.

Termination of treatment. Every effort should be made to finish treatment with the patient in good spirits and enthusiastic about returning for further treatment. Attention to him should take preference over straightening-up activities that could be done when he has left.

Other types of treatment. Although the prescription only calls for massage, permission should be sought to preheat the limb and combine stretching and active exercise to the physical therapy program. This boy could also profit from occupational therapy to encourage functional re-education for the entire arm and hand.

How to tell if objectives have been accomplished

If range of motion increases (determined by goniometer measurements compared with first day), the major objective of treatment has been accomplished. If the boy relaxes and cooperates with the program, treatment will be more effective. If the boy continues to improve in the functional use of his arm, it can be assumed that treatment is accomplishing the objectives for which it was designed. If no increase in range of motion is noticeable, he should be referred back to his doctor.

Summary

This is an example illustrating how these cases may be worked out. Every therapist will think of different ways to do it. Regardless of how it is done, the experience of working it out for oneself is where the real value of such an exercise lies.

Cases

1

Diagnosis
This three-year-old boy has received a severe burn to the right wrist. There is extensive scar tissue and flexion contractures at the wrist joint.

Treatment
Massage to the right forearm and hand in preparation for stretching.

2

Diagnosis
This fifty-year-old woman has hypertension and is unable to sleep.

Treatment
Back massage to encourage relaxation.

3

Diagnosis

This twenty-year-old male's right shoulder and arm have just been removed from cast because of surgery to relieve recurrent shoulder dislocation.

Treatment

Give tapotement, effleurage, and petrissage to deltoid and trapezius in an attempt to increase circulation and relieve spasm.

4

Diagnosis

This railroad worker lost his left foot when he fell beneath a train six weeks ago. Surgical repair has been done and a stump seven inches below the knee remains. There are flexion contractures at the knee.

Treatment

Give massage to the left leg, including gentle to increasing percussion to the stump end.

5

Diagnosis

This fifty-five-year-old taxi driver has had severe bursitis in the right shoulder for two years.

Treatment

Give heat, massage, and exercise to the right shoulder.

6

Diagnosis

This football player suffered a torn semilunar cartilage in last week's game. The knee is swollen and tender. He cannot bear weight on it.

Treatment

Very light massage to reduce spasm and pain.

7

Diagnosis

This forty-three-year-old woman suffered amputation of the left breast two weeks ago due to a malignant tumor. The shoulder is painful and motion is limited.

Treatment

Massage to relieve pain and increase motion.

8

Diagnosis

This truck driver crushed his foot, receiving multiple fractures, eight weeks ago. The foot is swollen and painful. Motion at the ankle joint is limited. Recent x-rays show all fractures have healed.

Treatment

Massage to reduce swelling, reduce pain, and increase motion of all joints involved. Preheat the part by using whirlpool at 110°F and follow massage with exercise.

9

Diagnosis

This paraplegic woman has developed a large decubitus ulcer over the sacrum.

Treatment

Massage surrounding tissues to stimulate circulation.

10

Diagnosis

This fifteen-year-old girl was in an automobile accident. She has a fractured right femur which confines her to bed, in traction. In addition to the femur there are fractures to the jaw and left elbow. She complains of severe pain in the back due to the uncomfortable position caused by traction to the leg.

Treatment
Give massage to the back. Please move this patient as little as possible.

11

Diagnosis
Onset of polio was diagnosed ten days ago in this ten-year-old boy. He has severe spasm of the hamstrings of both legs.

Treatment
Hot pack and massage both lower extremities.

12

Diagnosis
This forty-year-old professor has severe low back pain from a herniated disc with severe sciatica associated. Any right leg movements which stretch the sciatic nerve are painful.

Treatment
Give petrissage to the low back.

13

Diagnosis
This boy received a greenstick fracture of the right ulna two weeks ago. The cast was removed two days ago.

Treatment
Give massage to the right arm.

14

Diagnosis
This patient was operated on for a herniated disc at the fourth cervical level one week ago. There is slight swelling in the area.

Treatment
Massage in attempt to reduce swelling and relieve associated muscle spasm.

15

Diagnosis

This thirty-five-year-old woman received a fracture of the right humerus six weeks ago. The cast has been removed. There is limitation of motion at the shoulder and the elbow. The skin is irritated and tender. Heat has been applied.

Treatment

Massage in preparation for passive motion of the arm and shoulder.

16

Diagnosis

This forty-three-year-old woman has a suspected tumor at the C-3 level.

Treatment

Give deep massage, both petrissage and tapotement.

17

Diagnosis

This forty-five-year-old laborer suffers with myositis of the right upper trapezius.

Treatment

Give heat and massage to relieve pain and relax spasm.

18

Diagnosis

This neuropsychiatric patient is twenty-five years old and in a manic depressive state.

Treatment

Give back massage for sedation.

19

Diagnosis

This patient has had severe arthritis of the whole body for the past fifteen years. There is marked limitation of motion in the left knee; no motion of the patella; and a flexion deformity of the knee at 145°.

Treatment
Give massage to mobilize the left knee.

20

Diagnosis
The cast has just been removed from a well-healed fracture of the right elbow of this eight-year-old boy.

Treatment
Massage and exercise to mobilize the joint and strengthen the muscles.

21

Diagnosis
This female, age fifty-seven, fell and dislocated her left shoulder four weeks ago. She carries her arm in an airplane splint. There is also a stretch injury to the brachial plexus.

Treatment
Massage the entire shoulder, arm, and hand, being careful not to change the position of the shoulder.

22

Diagnosis
This thirty-year-old concert pianist suffers from chronic tenosynovitis of the middle finger of the left hand.

Treatment
Give paraffin bath to be followed by massage.

23

Diagnosis
This college basketball player sprained his ankle yesterday. There is considerable swelling; much pain exists.

Treatment

Massage in attempt to decrease swelling and get this player back into the game as soon as possible.

24

Diagnosis

This boy's elbow was hyperextended when he fell while ice skating, causing some tearing of the ligaments. Extention to 150° elicits pain. There is slight swelling and discoloration; the elbow is still tender.

Treatment

Heat has been applied. Massage in attempt to reduce swelling and alleviate pain.

25

Diagnosis

This young female patient has had acute myositis of the left tibialis anterior since an automobile accident about a year ago. There remains an area of "hardness" in the midshin region which limits the contracting range of the muscle.

Treatment

Massage to increase range of motion of the ankle joint.

26

Diagnosis

This fifty-year-old bricklayer has a chronic low back pain from an old lumbosacral strain.

Treatment

Massage.

27

Diagnosis

This fifty-year-old man has Bell's palsy on the right side following surgery for removal of a nonmalignant tumor of the parotid gland.

Treatment
Massage.

28

Diagnosis
This physical therapy school director has been having tension head-
aches involving spasm of the muscles of the upper back and neck,
especially on the right side.

Treatment
Massage to relieve tension in upper back and neck.

29

Diagnosis
This eighteen-year-old boy has a "baseball finger," index finger of
the right hand, with a chip fracture of the metacarpophalangeal
joint. There is pain and swelling.

Treatment
Give heat, massage, and active exercise.

30

Diagnosis
A gunshot wound was received when this thirty-year-old man was
cleaning his rifle. A twenty-two caliber bullet entered the body just
below the right clavicle and emerged through the right scapula,
shattering that bone and piercing the brachial plexus. The patient
was injured six months ago and there has been no return of innervation from the peripheral nerves damaged. He carries his arm close
to his body in a sling and complains of pain throughout the entire
shoulder and arm.

Treatment
Give heat, and massage prior to faradic muscle testing.

31

Diagnosis

This twenty-five-year-old butcher cut his arm just below the right elbow. The ulnar nerve injury had surgical repair two weeks ago.

Treatment

Give massage to the right lower arm and hand to increase circulation. Caution! Do not extend the elbow.

32

Diagnosis

This sixty-year-old man has had arthritis of the spine. He stands in a slightly flexed position. Extension to normal standing position produces pain.

Treatment

Heat and massage to relieve pain and spasm.

33

Diagnosis

This twenty-five-year-old secretary has a cervical rib which causes peripheral neuritis of the right upper extremity.

Treatment

Massage to relieve pain.

34

Diagnosis

This sixteen-year-old girl has a fracture of the neck of the right humerus following an automobile accident. She has been out of cast for two days. There is little range of motion of the shoulder, elbow, wrist, or hand. There is swelling and pain.

Treatment

Massage in preparation for mobilization.

35

Diagnosis

This normal twenty-year-old male is a star member of his college football team. Whether his team can win tomorrow will depend a great deal on how fast he can run and how far he can kick.

Treatment

Massage to precondition this player for peak performance the following day.

36

Diagnosis

Casting has just been removed from this four-year-old girl to correct bilaterally, congenitally dislocated hips.

Treatment

Use whirlpool followed by massage.

37

Diagnosis

This ten-year-old girl fell on the way home from the grocery store, breaking a bottle of milk and severely cutting the thenar eminance of her right hand on the broken fragments of glass. Tendon repair was done ten days ago.

Treatment

Very cautiously massage, precede with heat, and follow with gentle active exercise.

38

Diagnosis

This press-punch operator has developed a severe subdeltoid bursitis which inhibits his capacity to work.

Treatment

Use ultrasound, massage, and exercise.

39

Diagnosis

This woman slipped going downstairs into the subway station, fracturing the posterior aspect of the right calcaneus, four weeks ago. She is suing the subway for injuries received which may be the factor accounting for her seeming reluctance to regain normal range of motion.

Treatment

Give massage and exercise.

40

Diagnosis

This young woman fell from a horse three weeks ago. She was wearing glasses with metal frames. As she was dragged, with one foot caught in the stirrup, her face was deeply cut, tearing it from the lateral aspect of the right eye toward the mouth. The formation of keloid causes more disfiguration than normal and some adhesions are beginning to develop.

Treatment

Massage to loosen peripheral, adhesive scar tissue. If keloid formation increases report to the doctor for possible use of x-ray.

41

Diagnosis

This patient is just recovering from a chemo-pallidectomy for Parkinson's disease on the right. The right hand is now free of spasm or tremor, but is stiff from disuse. The finger flexors remain tight and the patient seems reluctant to try using his hand for daily activities.

Treatment

Give heat, massage, and exercise to assist the patient in regaining use of the hand.

42

Diagnosis

This patient has hysterical paralysis of both lower extremities following real but nonparalytic polio. His younger sister suffers from
paralysis of both lower extremities following polio just previous to
the onset of her brothers.

Treatment

Give heat, massage, and exercise to support psychotherapy. This
patient is to be approached by the therapist exactly as if his paralysis
were real. Any sign of muscle re-education should be enthusiastically
encouraged.

43

Diagnosis

This twenty-one-year-old man had a triple arthrodesis four weeks
ago for correction of a club foot.

Treatment

Massage in preparation for mobilization of foot.

44

Diagnosis

This eighty-five-year-old woman had a cup arthroplasty of the right
hip one week ago, following a nonunion fracture of the head of the
femur.

Treatment

Give heat, massage, and exercise to the right hip.

45

Diagnosis

All fingers of the left hand of this twenty-seven-year-old housewife
were crushed in the car door of the family station wagon. There
were multiple fractures of all fingers across the tips, with some chip

fractures into the first joint. The nail of the middle finger is off and those of the others in various stages of recovery.

Treatment

Massage the left hand, especially the fingers, in preparation for exercise to regain normal function of the hand.

In areas where students are able to work with patients early in their specialized education, cases which they are treating can be written up. The following outline * may be used:

A. Case History (to include the following):
    1. Present date
    2. Age, sex, and race of patient
    3. Diagnosis and pathology (also contributing factors or complications, if any)
    4. Significant dates (onset, surgery, casts, etc.)
    5. Type of patient (wheel chair, crutches, ambulatory, etc.; distinguish between hospitalized and out-patients)
B. Treatment ordered (mention all treatment ordered but elaborate only on massage)
    1. Type of treatment
    2. Frequency of treatment
C. Precautions
D. Positioning
    1. General position (sitting, lying supine, prone, etc.)
    2. Support indicated (pillows, etc.)
    3. Is elevation indicated?
E. Draping
F. Type of lubrication
G. Organization of routine (including amount of pressure used)
H. Duration of entire massage treatment (indicate approximately how time would be proportioned)
I. Termination
J. Source of information for history and treatment

* This outline was created by Vera Kaska, Instructor of Massage, University of Connecticut School of Physical Therapy. It is reproduced here with her permission.

Summary

No one student can do justice to the consideration of all these cases! Certain ones can be assigned while others can be used for open discussion in class. Others can be used in laboratory practice sessions. Any use made of them will increase the ability of the students to meet and solve problems similar to those they will soon be facing in the clinical areas. These cases will not be useful to those in the field of athletics or nursing. Therefore the special uses of massage in these two fields will be discussed in the next two chapters.

14

Use of Massage in Athletics

The well-rounded training program of any physical education major should include massage. The coach should know how to make use of massage for conditioning *before* activity and following extreme activity to prevent or reduce lameness. This does not mean that all the members of whatever team he might be coaching could be given conditioning massage before every game.

There are apt to be instances when such use of massage might make the difference between breaking a record by some outstanding member of the track team or swimming event. In cases such as this, massage might add just enough by way of extra nourishment to the vital muscle groups to make this extra effort well worth the coach's time.

Massage for conditioning before extreme activity
The following treatment should be given the day *before* the expected activity. The athlete should plan on a half hour of complete rest following this treatment and an evening which insures minimal exertion and a good night of sleep.

Massage should be preceded by a brisk needle shower which works from warm (about 110°) to cool (about 80°).

With the person lying prone, give a general brief massage which covers the back, working from light effleurage rather quickly into deep effleurage and petrissage of all the large muscle groups of the back. Encourage relaxation and make sure that the resting position is comfortable.

When sufficient general relaxation has been obtained, massage can be begun on the muscle groups which will be used most with the activity planned for the coming day. Thus, if the event requires running, the legs would be carefully massaged with deep effleurage of the gluteals, hamstrings and gastrocnemii, working to deep kneading of all these muscle groups, not forgetting the anterior aspects of the leg, particularly the quadriceps and anterior tibial group.

When each muscle group has been carefully massaged, the whole extremity should be gone over again with long sweeping effleurage strokes which follow from the heel all the way up the back of the leg and over the gluteals.

Brisk tapotement of any type leaves the patient with a feeling of tingling well-being.

In the same manner, if the coming event will involve the arms, the latter part of the massage considers mostly the thoracic spine and arms. If the activity involves the use of all four extremities, the total body should be considered, doing first one side and then the other.

Although there are probably no statistics to prove this theory, those who have had experience have come to realize the value of putting essential muscle groups into a good metabolic state previous to extremes of activity. There is less tendency toward Charley horse with such conditioning and less tendency toward lameness following such activity.

This concept is far from being a new one. It has been done since the days of ancient Roman gladiators.

Massage following extreme activity

Whereas the purpose of preconditioning is to ready the muscles for exertion, the purpose of massage following such activity is to carry away the waste products which have collected due to this exertion. It does not require stimulation, for the muscle has been stimulated and is now tired and seeking rest and inactivity. If the muscle is exhausted enough, it will not perform its normal activity of "milking" these by-products into the venous return. The person who has put forth a supreme effort is physically tired, and at this stage of the game exercise cannot accomplish the desired exchange in metabolism because the muscles themselves are too weary to profit by further exercise.

Therefore the purpose at this point is to "wring out" the muscle and mechanically do this job of milking for it. Gently kneading the muscle free of such by-products will allow it to take advantage of the fresh supply of blood and lymph which automatically follows the massage.

Since stimulation is not desired, a warm shower should precede the massage. The rate of the stroke is much slower. (Remember the flow of lymph is slow and sluggish.) Watch the more superficial veins and give them time to refill following the effleurage stroke. If muscle soreness is involved, pressure must be regulated so that it is firm enough to squeeze out the muscle without provoking a "muscle splinting" type of protective tensing.

Tapotement is not indicated unless the individual requests it, for now the aim is not one of stimulation or preparation but rather rest and complete relaxation, which in itself allows a normal return of new and nourishing blood to the tired muscle and minimizes the tightness and spasm that come from stiff and sore muscles.

If any tightness or spasm is present, and there is no injury to the muscle, such as rupture or hematoma, active normal range of motion may be attempted. If there has been any sign of injury to the muscle, no treatment of any kind should be attempted without consultation with a physician.

Charley horse (muscle cramp or spasm)

If a muscle is asked to do more than it has been "conditioned" to do, and extreme activity is undertaken without proper warm-up exercises or a building-up to be able to do a task of sudden activity, the result will be sudden, painful spasm of the muscle. The muscle is not able to meet the chemical exchanges to keep its metabolic balance.

The name *Charley horse* has also been given to the painful spasm that results from severe kicks or blows, which are accidentally received in competitive activity.

Upon occasion the muscle will actually rupture and hematoma can readily be seen. If there is any indication that these spasms or cramps have been severe enough to cause bleeding within the muscle belly or tearing of the tendon, no measures should be taken to massage or exercise the part until advised to do so by a physician.

If, however, there is cramping due to inability of the muscle to meet the metabolic needs and stresses placed upon it, effleurage and petrissage can assist the muscle back to normalcy. If the muscles do go into spasm, it is an indication that these muscles are not in condition for activity. Conditioning exercises will avoid repetition of such "casualties."

Summary

General knowledge of all the massage techniques will be valuable information for those in the field of physical education. Judicious and ethical precautions should be taken to avoid treating any injury that should not be treated by massage. The major uses of massage in athletics as set forth in this brief chapter will lessen chances of injury, prevent unnecessary lameness, and prepare muscles for peak performance.

15

The Use of Massage in Nursing

Traditionally the nurse has given massage as part of the daily care of the patient. Patients confined to bed develop areas of discomfort due simply to inactivity. Chapter 4, Part I explains the physiological reasons for this discomfort and tells how massage can relieve this type of distress.

Many schools are placing increased emphasis on massage because they realize how this valuable tool can comfort the distraught patient, both physically and psychologically. Massage is one of the key points of good nursing care. It produces a permissive atmosphere for communication between nurse and patient. It creates a situation in which the patient literally *feels* the interest and concern of the nurse for his welfare.

With skillful hands the nurse can gain the confidence of her patients. At the same time discomfort can quickly and easily be relieved through the physiological, mechanical, and reflex effects of massage. Such a massage need not take more than five minutes. In fact, the patient who is ill enough to be confined to bed will tire quickly. More than five minutes may do more harm than good.

Any or all of the techniques described may be used. There is seldom need for tapotement, but if its stimulating effects are desired it could be used without harm to the patient.

Massage of normal tissue, which is not involved with the patient's pathological condition, can often relax him when he is restless from long hours in bed. Nurses who can skillfully execute basic massage techniques will earn the gratitude of their patients, particularly under the circumstances described in this chapter.

Massage of the back

Any time the patient has been lying on his back for quite a while, massage to the back is recommended. In preparing the patient for rest and sleep, the entire massage should be done in a slow, rhythmical, relaxed fashion. This contact presents an excellent time to build confidence in the patient and promote feelings of security and well-being. Empathy can be shown without words. A soothing voice, combined with light rhythmical stroking, can strongly motivate the patient toward restful sleep.

There is often muscular tightness through the shoulder and neck muscles due to uncomfortable positions and increased tension of the patient. Strong petrissage to this area can relieve such tightness.

In concluding, strokes should work from deep to light. Strokes which go downward from the head toward the coccyx are more restful than those which go upward. The relaxing stroke described on page 50 will often leave the patient almost asleep.

Massage for pressure areas

All patients who lie quietly in bed, due to paralysis or weakness, should receive good massage to areas where pressure is apt to cause decubitus ulcers. Combined with frequent changes of position and proper resting positions, massage can help prevent their formation.

Deep strokes which bring blood to the area should be applied each time the patient is moved. Here again, this need not take a great deal of time, but the results will be most gratifying.

Common sites for decubitus ulcers are over the sacrum, the back of the heels, elbows, and knees. When the patient is turned one can readily see where pressure has recently been placed. Effleurage and petrissage may be applied with depth. Stroking *toward* the pressure area will encourage capillary dilatation. Friction can also be applied around the pressure area. Once a decubitus ulcer has developed to an acute phase, massage alone will be of little use and should not be attempted by the nurse.

Massage for the immobilized patient

Patients who have been immobilized by traction or casts often become very uncomfortable because of positions that must be maintained. The patient with a leg in traction may complain that his back or his neck is uncomfortable.

With precaution against moving the injured limb, massage to the uncomfortable area can relieve much of this type of discomfort.

Teamwork between nursing and physical therapy

Many times the duties of these two professions overlap. Massage is one of the areas where the nurse might wonder when to do it herself, and when to refer the patient to the physical therapy department. Since strong emphasis is placed on having both nurses and physical therapists work under the specific prescription of the doctor, care must be taken not to violate this ethical regulation. Massage to *healthy tissue* for the relief of discomfort could bring little harm to the patient. If at any time there is doubt as to whether a technique should be used, the nurse will protect her patient by checking with the doctor before proceeding. There are times when the nurse, working closely with the physical therapist and the doctor, can supplement the massage done by the physical therapist. This is true more often when a private duty nurse has the time for this type of treatment.

Summary

The nurse with trained and sensitive hands can greatly relieve minor discomforts of the patient without feeling that she is overstepping the bounds of her profession. It takes little time and means a great deal to the patient. Massage is valuable for more than the mechanical and physiological effects mentioned in this chapter. The psychological effect of this close attention should not be underestimated.

Recommended Reading for Part II

Barnett, E. M.: Mimeographed Report, Sargent School of Physical Therapy.

Copestake, B. M. G.: *The Theory and Practice of Massage,* 4th ed. Paul B. Hoeber, Inc., New York, 1926, Chapters XI–XIII.

Cyriax, James: *Treatment by Manipulation and Deep Massage,* 6th ed. Paul B. Hoeber, Inc., New York, 1959.

Dicke, Elisabeth: *Meine Bindegewebsmassage.* Hippokrates-Verlag, Stuttgart, 1956.

Graham, Douglas: *Massage Manual Treatment and Remedial Movements,* 4th. ed. J. B. Lippincott Co., Philadelphia, 1913, Chapters V–XXVIII.

Hoffa, Albert J.: *Technik der Massage,* 3rd ed. Ferdinand Enke, Stuttgart, 1900.

McMillan, Mary: *Massage and Therapeutic Exercise,* 3rd. ed. W. B. Saunders Co., Philadelphia, 1932, pp. 17–41.

Mennell, James B.: *Physical Treatment by Movement, Manipulation and Massage,* 4th ed. The Blakiston Co., Philadelphia, 1940, Chapters III–XXXV.

Nissen, Hartvig: *Practical Massage and Corrective Exercises.* F. A. Davis Co., Philadelphia, 1939, Chapters XIX–XXVIII.

Storms, Harold D.: "Diagnostic and Therapeutic Massage," *Arch. of Phys. Med.,* Vol. XXV, (Sept.) 1944, pp. 550–52.

Tidy, Noel M.: *Massage and Remedial Exercises,* 4th ed. Williams and Wilkins, Baltimore, 1939.

III

Variations of Massage Techniques

16

Albert J. Hoffa

This discussion does not include the *complete* translation of Hoffa's text for much of it would not be applicable today. However a complete translation has been made and the techniques described here closely follow the literal translation.*

Hoffa uses what he describes as the anatomical method for the different parts of the body, following the larger vessels, and selecting specific muscles or muscle groups to be massaged in order.

He states that the following general considerations should be kept in mind. The force should not be rude or brutal and all manipulations should be gentle and "light-handed" so that the patient feels as little pain as possible. No point should be treated for too long. Hoffa's text does not advocate any massage for over fifteen minutes, even for a total body massage.†

No massage should be done through clothing. The part to be massaged should be as relaxed as possible. The joints should be kept in mid-position so that tension of capsule ligaments and tendons are at a minimum.

---

* With the help of Miss Ruth Friedlander, the author translated Hoffa's book into English. Passages quoted in this chapter are from that translation, but the page numbers refer to Hoffa's text in case the reader should wish to refer to the original.

† Max Bohm's book (*Massage: Its Principles and Technic,* translated by Elizabeth Gould. W. B. Saunders Co., Philadelphia, 1913) which is representative of Hoffa's technique as interpreted by Bohm, states, however, that up to three-quarters of an hour can be taken for massage of the whole body.

If the hands are rough a lubricant should be used. Hoffa states that if the part to be massaged is covered with hair it should be shaved. The therapist should start with the healthy part and massage gradually toward the injured area, always stroking with the venous flow.

Effleurage should be used for beginning and ending the massage as well as between all other strokes. If the part is covered by thick heavy fascia, effleurage is not deep enough and greater pressure is needed. Therefore, the knuckles must be used. Pressure is not continuous, but swells up and down, starting lightly and becoming stronger, then decreasing again. The hand should not stick to the part but glide over it lightly. If the hands are moist, they should be washed with alcohol and rubbed with salicylic powder.

Hoffa's Effleurage Techniques

Light and deep stroking

The following description of effleurage is applied to both light and deep stroking; the deep stroking differs only in the amount of pressure applied:

> The hand is applied as closely as possible to the part. It glides on it, distally to proximally. . . . With the broad part of the hand use the ball of the thumb and little fingers to stroke out the muscle masses, and at the same time, slide along at the edge of the muscle with finger tips to take care of all larger vessels; stroke upward (Hoffa, p. 2).

Knuckling

Knuckling is a stroke particularly associated with the techniques of Hoffa. In describing it he says:

> If the part to be treated is covered by thick fascia, effleurage (as described above) is not deep enough. You need greater pressure, therefore the convex dorsal sides of the first interphalangeal joints must be used. Clench the fist in strong plantar flexion, knuckles in the peripheral end stroking upwards, by gradually bringing the hand from plantar to dorsal

flexion. Pressure is not continuous, swelling up and down, starting lightly
and becoming stronger, then decreasing again. The hand must not adhere
to the part, but should glide over it lightly. Knuckling should only be used
where there is enough room for the hand to be applied (Hoffa, p. 2).

Circular effleurage

Hoffa often refers to what he calls "circular effleurage." In regard
to circular effleurage of the fingers he writes:

> To do circular effleurage of each single finger, stroke around each finger
> from its point to its base, with strokes that cover each other like the
> shingles of a roof. Execute these strokes with the tip of the index and
> middle finger of the right hand, held in opposition to each other, while
> you lay the volar surface on your own left hand underneath the fingers
> on which you are working to support them. To make this stroke more
> vigorous use the tips of your two thumbs (Hoffa, p. 51).

Adapting circular effleurage to the arm, he describes it saying,
"Begin on the forearm, stroking around the joint and doing strokes
in such a manner that they always end up in either the biceps or
triceps group. While one hand supports, the other hand massages"
(Hoffa, p. 58).

Thumb stroking

Hoffa uses an alternate thumb stroking on the foot. He describes its
use on the dorsum of the foot by saying, "Massage each tendon
sheath by means of strokes of the thumb, alternating from the base
of the toes up over the ankle joint" (Hoffa, p. 62).

Alternate hand stroking

No description of alternate effleurage stroking could be found other
than the use of alternate *thumb* stroking on the foot.

Others

Hoffa mentions the use of simultaneous stroking and the use of one-
hand stroking, but does not describe the use of the one hand over
the other for deeper pressure (Hoffa, pp. 29, 32).

Hoffa's Petrissage Techniques

One-hand petrissage

Place the hand around the part so that the muscle-masses are caught between the fingers and thumb as in a pair of tongs. By lifting the muscle-mass from the bone, "squeeze them out," progressing centripetally. On flat surfaces where this petrissage is not possible, Hoffa does a stroke using a flat hand instead of picking up the muscle. This type of kneading is recommended for use on small limbs (Hoffa, p. 9).

Two-hand petrissage

Apply both hands obliquely to the direction of the muscle fibers. The thumbs are opposed to the rest of the fingers. This manipulation starts peripherally and proceeds centripetally, following the direction of the muscle fibers. The hand that goes first tries to pick the muscle from the bone, moving back and forth in a zigzag path. The hand that follows proceeds likewise, "gripping back and forth." This progressive movement is made easier by doing most of the work from the shoulder (Hoffa, pp. 9–10). On flat surfaces where this petrissage is not possible Hoffa does the stroke using a *flat* hand, instead of picking up the muscle.

Two-finger petrissage

Over parts where muscle bellies are flat rather than round, and one cannot grasp hold with a full hand (such as the back, or over places where muscles are overlaid by strong fascias) the most useful kind of petrissage is the two-finger petrissage. Grasp the part between thumb and forefinger. Press it out by making little circular movements from the shoulder, making the fingers move the skin along with the rest of the movement. Some people refer to this as "creepy crawl" or "creepy mouse," but neither term connotes relaxation. This author prefers Hoffa's terminology, "two-finger petrissage."

Friction

In describing friction Hoffa says:

> Put the thumb in the neighborhood of the part to be massaged, setting the index finger of the right hand on the skin of the part, more or less vertically. Penetrate into the depth, not by moving the points of the fingers on the skin, but by moving the skin under the fingers.
>
> In going deep, describe small flat ellipsoids with the point of the index finger. These follow each other as quickly and consecutively as possible. The finger joints and wrist are to be kept almost stiff and the elbow joint only makes small excursions. The main movement is made from the shoulder joint (Hoffa, pp. 11–12).

He uses the finger of the left hand to intersperse effleurage with the friction strokes.

In reference to the use of other fingers or parts of the hand for friction, Hoffa refers only to the thumb, using it either to fit better to some anatomical part or to rest the forefinger. He also suggests using both thumb and index finger to do friction at the same time.

Hoffa uses the *thumb*, the *index finger, or both* for friction.

Tapotement

In describing tapotement, Hoffa says, "Both hands are held vertically above the part to be treated in a position that is midway between pronation and supination. Bringing them into supination, the abducted fingers are hit against the body with not too much force and with great speed and elasticity. Fingers and wrists remain as stiff as possible but the shoulder joint comes into play all the more actively" (Hoffa, p. 14). Hoffa used this hacking stroke routinely with all back massages.

Vibration

Hoffa says that vibration may be done either with the points of the fingers or with the hand lying flat. The forearm is at right angles to the upper arm. The whole forearm is brought into a rhythmical trembling movement from the elbow joint, but the wrist and finger joints are kept as stiff as possible. Even though he describes the technique, he feels that it is better to use a mechanical vibrator (Hoffa, pp. 15, 17).

Massage of the upper extremity

In describing stroking and petrissage of the limbs, Hoffa begins with the right forearm, dividing it into two groups, the flexors and the extensors. The hand and foot are discussed separately. The patient sits facing the therapist, with the arm in a neutral position between flexion and abduction, and the elbow at an obtuse angle with the radial side upward. The patient should be as relaxed as possible. Three or four times is enough of each stroke to accomplish the purpose of effleurage.

After stroking out the muscles, petrissage is given. As in effleurage the muscle groups should be kept strictly in mind. First the extensors are kneaded, starting at the wrist and ending at the elbow. The hand of the therapist lifts up the extensors between the thumb and the other four fingers, kneading them centripetally. Once having arrived at the elbow joint, a few effleurage strokes are interspersed about three times before kneading of the flexors is undertaken in a similar manner.

The upper arm is divided into three muscle groups. Group one includes the biceps, brachialis and coracobrachialis. The second group is the triceps muscle alone; the third division is the deltoid, which is divided into two parts, the back and the front. Massage of the upper arm begins with the stroking and kneading of the biceps group. The triceps are then considered. The therapist applies her hand to the back of the arm, beginning just below the olecranon, gliding upward in the external bicipital sulcus and then on to the outer edge of the deltoid and into the auxilliary pit. The posterior part of the deltoid is massaged before the anterior portion and the massage to the upper extremity is finished.

In massage of the hand, Hoffa does a circular effleurage of each of the fingers. In doing this he strokes around each finger from its point to its base with strokes that cover each other like the shingles of a roof. He executes these strokes with the tip of the index and middle finger of the right hand, held in opposition to each other, while he lays the volar surface of his own left hand underneath the fingers on which he is working to support them. These strokes he refers to as "shingle strokes" (Hoffa, pp. 23–62).

For petrissage of the fingers, he takes hold of the soft part from both sides between the thumb and forefinger of his two hands and picks them up off the bone (as best he can), while moving along the skin and describing small circles, squeezing and progressing from the point of one finger to the base of the other in a zigzag fashion. The rest of the hand is done with alternate thumb stroking from the metacarpophalangeal joint to the wrist and knuckling is done to the palmar fascia. The massage of the foot is very similar (Hoffa, pp. 51–62).

Massage of the lower extremity

Hoffa mentions turning the patient when treating both front and back of the lower extremity. (This technique is no longer widely practiced and it is felt that the patient should not be disturbed any more than is absolutely necessary.) The therapist should place the patient either on his back or prone and adapt all techniques so that anterior and posterior aspects of the lower extremity are treated from one position.

Hoffa shows an illustration of the patient seated, with his leg in the therapist's lap (Hoffa, p. 23). This author doubts that Hoffa, were he alive today, would recommend a position where support of the limb is so poor.

For massage of the lower extremity, the patient is seated, with his leg in the therapist's lap (Hoffa, p. 23). The hip is in inward rotation, the knee slightly bent for massage of the outer muscles, and the leg is rotated outward to reach the medial muscle groups.

Beginning with the lower leg, he divides it into four groups: first, the tibialis anticus with the extensors digitorum, communis longus, and hallucis longus; second, the peroneal muscles; third, the outer half of the calf muscles; fourth, the inner half of the calf muscles with the tibialis posticus, flexor hallucis longus and flexor digitorum communis longus. Taking the above named groups in order, they are effleuraged and petrissaged. On the first group the usual effleurage is followed by a few strokes done with the knuckles, due to the strong crural fascia. Two-finger petrissage is also used on this group. At the knee joint the therapist intersperses a few effleurage strokes and begins to knead again. The peroneal group is covered in like manner. The last two groups are massaged with the usual effleurage and one-hand petrissage.

Massage of the thigh is divided into the quadriceps, adductors, tensor fascia lata, biceps, semitendinosus and semimembranosus and the glutei. For massage of the quadriceps and adductor group the patient lies on his back, and for the tensor fascia lata he lies on his side. For the remaining parts he lies on his stomach. All groups are given effleurage and petrissage in the prescribed manner, with knuckling over the tensor fascia lata. The glutei are divided into two groups, considering the oblique direction of the fibers that run from the trochanter towards the iliac crest and those from the greater trochanter toward the sacrum and then toward the iliac crest. The therapist is seated on the side of the patient opposite that which she is massaging. Both sections are given effleurage and petrissage.

Massage of the back

The back massage first considers the long, back muscles, with the stroke beginning at the limit between the back and neck. The stroke

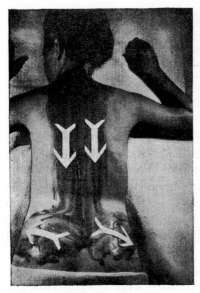
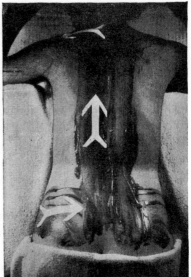

Figure 43
Erector spinae group.

Figure 44
Erector spinae group.

progresses downward, leaving the spinous processes free, with the tips of the first and second fingers performing most of the stroke (Fig. 43). As the hands reach the sacrum, they diverge laterally from each other and follow the course of the iliac crest to the inguinal region. There the stroke is ended and the upward stroke begins. The stroke returns in a similar fashion to the sacrum and proceeds upward to the hairline (Fig. 44) where the hands glide along the neck laterally to arrive at the sternoclavicular joint. After several repetitions of these strokes, the therapist follows it with knuckle effleurage to affect the deeper tissues. Two-finger petrissage is then given to the long muscles of the back. The fingerpaint patterns illustrate direction of the strokes and the area covered.

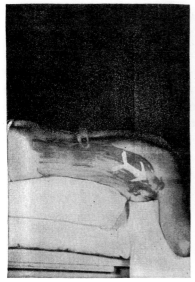

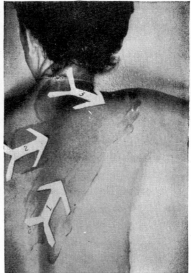

Figure 45
Latissimus dorsi.

Figure 46
Trapezius.

The latissimus dorsi is then effleuraged from origin to insertion (Fig. 45). The trapezius is divided into three groups in accordance with the three-fold fiber direction (Fig. 46). Each group is considered separately and given effleurage. This is contrary to the common opinion that Hoffa stroked the trapezius with an alternate effleurage stroke, but the description given here is upheld by Bohm (Bohm, p. 73). Petrissage, using the flat hand, is given on the latissimus dorsi and lower and middle trapezius. Tapotement in the form of hacking is given after all muscle groups have been effleuraged and petrissaged. All of one side of the back is done before the therapist goes to the opposite side of the table and does the opposite side of the back.

Summary

The fact that Hoffa was one of the earliest to describe massage in a text, coupled with the accuracy of his descriptions, may account for the fact that his five fundamental strokes are still done today much as they were then, although the pattern or area of the stroke may vary greatly. Principles of positioning have changed since the days when Hoffa put the patient's foot comfortably in his lap to work on it! There is no denying that Hoffa's methods are still used throughout America today, although the therapists using them are often unaware that they were ever written in German by Hoffa. It is hoped this text will enlighten many and give Hoffa the credit that is most certainly due him.

17

Mary McMillan

Mary McMillan considers massage as manipulation of soft tissues or as movements done upon the body. She divides massage into five fundamental procedures: effleurage, petrissage, friction, tapotement, and vibration. She also organizes her discussion of massage in that order.

She feels that the student beginning to use her hands in various forms of manipulation has little difficulty in getting accustomed to dry rubbing. Miss McMillan prefers it, except in cases of excessive scar tissue, or for very emaciated patients, or after the long use of splints. She feels that cod liver oil, or olive oil, can be of nutritive value when absorbed through the pores of the skin and would therefore be a good lubricant to use if this type of nutrition is desired. Cocoa butter and lanolin are among the best lubricants, but should be used sparingly. The latter is preferred by some because it is an animal fat.

Miss McMillan's massage was developed from her experience in teaching. Although it is not based on a particular method, she makes reference to J. M. M. Lucas-Championnière, Sir William Bennett, Dr. Weir Mitchell, and Dr. Douglas Graham.

She believes that a definite amount of body surface should be decided upon before the hand begins the stroke.

For example, thorough stroking of the whole arm involves the following operations: First, from the finger-tips to just beyond the wrist-joint; second, from below the wrist-joint to just beyond the elbow-joint; third, from below the elbow-joint to just beyond the shoulder-joint.

It will be noticed in each subdivision that the stroke is carried from just below the distal joint to just beyond the proximal, the object being to carry the lymph to the proximal glands in order that it may be taken on through the lymphatics, back to the right side of the heart.

An operator who cannot use one hand as well as the other is not only limited in performing the normal operations of the work, but is a 50 per cent worker. Therefore, from the start, one should practice more with the lesser developed hand as soon as some ability to perform certain manipulations is acquired. Great care should be taken to put pressure on the upward stroke, allowing the hand to return to its original position without pressure, but without losing contact with the part being massaged. The fingers of the operator in performing effleurage should be held close together, but not stiffly. Relaxation on the part of the patient is necessary. The greater the facility of the operator to mold the hand into the part being massaged, the better the work will be. This molding is making use to the utmost advantage of the span between the thumb and the fingers *en masse.* Most of the molding process is directed by the thumb and the thenar eminence. No jarring or jerking either at the start or finish of the stroke should ever be felt by the patient.°

Concerning treatment time and draping Miss McMillan says:

. . . There is no hard-and-fast rule, but the following table, stating the approximate length of time for the limbs and trunk, is given as an aid to beginners:

Upper limbs	10 minutes
Lower limbs	15 "
Back	7 "
Chest	5 "
Abdomen	5 "

. . . There is no need of exposing any part of the body other than that under treatment at the time. If there is any danger of the patient's taking cold, massage may be given under . . . a light-weight covering. If the patient wears a night-gown, each arm should be taken from the sleeve and replaced when treated. A light-weight but warm shawl is useful to cover the upper part of the back while the lower part is being massaged.†

° Mary McMillan: *Massage and Therapeutic Exercise,* 3rd ed. W. B. Saunders Co., Philadelphia, 1932, pp. 20–21.
† *Ibid.,* pp. 66–67.

Joint surfaces

Around joint surfaces pressure is brought to bear upon the underlying structures. In friction of the phalangeal joints the joints of the first and third fingers are manipulated between the finger and thumb of the operator. In the same way the second and fourth fingers receive friction. If friction is given simultaneously to alternate fingers, one hand of the operator is not in the way of the other. Friction is given around the wrist-joint with two or three fingers and thumb. In the lower extremity the toes and ankle-joint receive similar treatment. In cases in which there is excessive scar tissue friction is the most useful form of manipulation to loosen it. . . .

Running frictions are sometimes used to advantage in a case of recovering sciatica. Over the denser area the thenar eminence is used for the circular frictions, starting over the great sciatic notch where the sciatic nerve emerges from the pelvis. These friction movements are carried down the whole area of the terminal endings of the sciatic nerve.[*]

McMillan's Effleurage Techniques

Light and deep effleurage

In describing effleurage, Miss McMillan uses the whole of the palmar surface of the hand. Although light, the stroke is firm and even. The pressure is upward. The fingers are together and the hand is molded to the part. Most of this molding process is directed by the thumb and thenar eminence (McMillan, p. 19).

Alternate-hand stroking

Concerning alternate-hand stroking, Miss McMillan says, "The third division of the lower extremity is the thigh. Here, because there is a larger surface to cover, it is well to stroke with alternate hands. . . . There should be about six alternate hand strokings over the posterior surface of the thigh . . ."[†]

[*] *Ibid.*, pp. 36–38.
[†] *Ibid.*, p. 25.

Others

Miss McMillan uses both *simultaneous stroking* and *one-hand stroking,* but does not make reference to the use of knuckling, thumb stroking, or one hand over the other for deeper pressure (McMillan, pp. 24, 26).

McMillan's Petrissage Techniques

One- or two-hand petrissage

"Petrissage or kneading may be performed either with the whole of the palmar surface of the hand or by fingers and thumb." *

Two-finger petrissage

"For picking up small muscles (as, for example, those of the face) the forefinger and thumb are used." †

Petrissage of the back

For petrissage of the back she says, "Each section in turn is petrissaged by a pressure of muscles against the ribs, or, in the lumbar region, upon the abdominal wall. These muscles cannot be picked up as those in the limbs. The whole of the palmar surface of the hand is brought into play, but not in a molding manner as for the limbs, because the contour of the surface is flat instead of rounded." ‡

Alternate one-hand petrissage

"A useful variation of petrissage may be accomplished by the flexors and extensors being grasped by alternate hands, and a wringing movement being performed." §

* McMillan, *op. cit.,* p. 31.
† *Ibid.,* p. 31.
‡ *Ibid.,* pp. 33–34.
§ *Ibid.,* p. 31.

Friction

Regarding friction McMillan says:

Friction, or circular friction, is that form of manipulation in which the tips of the fingers or the fingers and thumbs are used—more especially around the bony prominences of joint surfaces. Pressure in a circular manner is brought to bear upon the underlying structures. This form of manipulation is extremely useful in breaking down adhesions and in promoting absorption. Friction should be followed by effleurage in order to send on through the blood-stream the broken-down products of inflammation.

Friction is performed by circular movements with the finger-tips, or with two or three finger-tips, or even with one, according to the amount of surface to be covered. . . . In friction of the phalangeal joints the joints of the first and third fingers are manipulated between the finger and thumb of the operator. In the same way the second and fourth fingers receive friction. . . .

Running frictions are sometimes used to advantage in a case of recovering sciatica. Over the denser area the thenar eminence is used for the circular frictions, starting over the great sciatic notch where the sciatic nerve emerges from the pelvis. These friction movements are carried down the whole area of the terminal endings of the sciatic nerve.[*]

Miss McMillan, then, uses the *thumb, two or three fingers, or the thenar eminence* for friction.

Tapotement

Tapotement is a series of brisk blows, one following another in rapid succession. It may be performed in four ways: Hacking, clapping, tapping, and beating.

Hacking is the most common form of tapotement. The operator's hands are held with ulnar borders of each ready to strike. The fingers are slightly flexed and parted, and the hands strike alternately. As the blow falls the fingers strike together. They are then separated, and the hand is raised some distance from the patient before the blow is repeated. Hacking is performed so as to strike transversely across the muscle-fibers from one end of the muscle to the other. . . .

Clapping is done with a cupped hand, the fingers and thumb being slightly flexed and the palmar surface contracted. This form of tapote-

[*] *Ibid.*, pp. 35–38.

ment is especially useful for covering the entire surface of the back. Clapping is also used over the chest muscles. It has a stimulating effect when used over peripheral vessels and nerves.

Tapping is performed with the fingers cone-shaped, and sharp, brisk tapping movements are applied with the tips to the surface desired. . . .

Beating is done with the ulnar border of the closed hand, as in making a fist. This form of tapotement is used over the gluteal muscles where the fascia is dense.*

Vibration

Vibration is performed with several fingers or even with one, and at times the whole palmar surface of the hand is used. A trembling sensation is conveyed by the operator . . .†

Massage of the upper extremity

In the first division of effleurage of the arm the palmar surface of the operator's hand supports the palmar surface of the patient's hand. The operator's working or active hand is then placed finger-tips to finger-tips with those of the patient; if the thumb-to-thumb method is adopted, it is much easier to fit hand to hand. Three or four firm, even strokings on the dorsal surface of the patient's hand are given. In order to conserve time and energy the operator, without changing hands, turns the patient's hand from the prone to the supine position; the supporting hand of the operator then becomes the active hand. The palmar surface is then stroked three or four times in a similar manner. In effleurage of the forearm the patient's hand is in the middle position between pronation and supination. One hand of the operator is used for the flexor group, while the other hand is supporting the part; then the hands should be reversed for the extensor group. The hands are now in position for effleurage of the upper arm, which is the third division. In a similar manner the flexor and extensor groups, each in turn, are stroked.‡

Miss McMillan then follows these same divisions, using petrissage and friction. She describes a useful variation of petrissage which

* *Ibid.*, pp. 38–40.

† *Ibid.*, p. 41.

‡ *Ibid.*, pp. 22–24.

may be used on both the flexors and the extensors. Grasping the flexors in one hand and the extensors in the other she performs an alternate wringing movement (McMillan, p. 31).

Massage of the lower extremity

In discussing massage of the lower extremity Miss McMillan states:

Subdivisions of the lower extremity correspond to those of the upper: First, foot; second, leg; third, thigh. In effleurage of the lower extremity the same procedure is used as with the upper extremity. The leg which is being massaged should never hang from the knee-joint, but should be well supported from the hip-joint.

The plantar surface of the foot from the tips of the toes to the heel is stroked with one hand. The other hand takes the stroke on the dorsal surface from the toes to beyond the ankle-joint. The whole palmar surface of the hand should conform to the sole of the foot.

The leg should be grasped with one hand covering the muscles on one side of the crest of the tibia, the other hand grasping the muscles on the other side. In this way one hand covers the anterior tibial group and the peroneal, while the other hand grasps the gastrocnemius group, the underlying and posterior tibial group being affected by the pressure from the superficial group. Always, where there are several layers of muscles, especially where the muscles are much developed, the stroking should be deeper, in order to reach the veins and lymphatic vessels which lie nearest the bone.

The third division of the lower extremity is the thigh. Here, because there is a larger surface to cover, it is well to stroke with alternate hands. At first both hands grasp the limb, finger-tips touching in the popliteal space, between inner and outer hamstring muscles. There should be about six alternate hand strokings over the posterior surface of the thigh, bringing the hands over the lateral aspects of the thigh to the anterior surface, where similar action is brought into play, until the whole of the thigh has been thoroughly stroked. This completes the general outline for effleurage of the limbs.*

Miss McMillan then follows these same divisions using petrissage and friction. Concerning petrissage she states:

The lower extremity also is divided into three divisions. The foot is petrissaged, special attention being paid to the muscles of the plantar

* *Ibid.,* pp. 24–26.

surface. The hand of the operator, making special use of the thenar eminence, kneads well into the plantar muscles. As the dorsum of the foot is so tendinous, petrissage is supplemented by running frictions between the interossei muscles. The spine of the tibia is used as a guide for the thumb of the operator in petrissage of the leg. On one side of the spine the muscles are kneaded by one hand, and on the other side of the spine by the other. If the small anterior tibial muscles require special care, finger-and-thumb petrissage is useful, as the muscle group is small and lies snugly against the tibia. In giving petrissage to the quadriceps group the two hands are used as one, the thumb of the right hand lying alongside the forefinger of the left hand, or vice versa. In this way the two hands, as one, pick up the anterior thigh muscles. The adductors and hamstrings are petrissaged by alternate hands.*

Massage of the back

It is well to divide the back into four main divisions, as there is so great an extent of surface. The patient should be in prone lying position on a straight plinth or bed with no pillows under the head. This position cannot be assumed by patients suffering from heart complication or from phthisis [tuberculosis] in which a hacking cough is aggravated by this position. In either of these cases, or when it is found inadvisable for the patient to lie flat, the back may be massaged while the patient is in a sitting posture. In general, however, the prone lying position is not at all uncomfortable for the majority of patients.

The first division of the back is from behind the ears, along the slope of the neck muscles, to the tip of the shoulder-girdle (Fig. 47). At the beginning of the stroke the forefinger is separated from the other fingers in order to get well behind the ears, and the stroke is carried until all the fingers come in close contact with each other again at the nape of the neck. With the same firm, even pressure, the stroke is then carried to its termination at the acromion process. In this division both hands of the operator start below the inferior angle of the scapulae and work in opposite directions from the center line, the stroke being repeated several times.

In the third division the hands start over the region of the sacrum and both hands stroke upward on corresponding sides until they reach the axilla. They are then brought back, one on each side of the trunk, each describing a circular movement. Care should be taken to cover the whole area with the upward stroke.

* *Ibid.,* pp. 32–33.

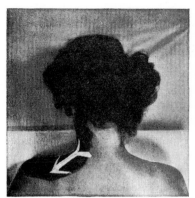

Figure 47
Upper trapezius, first division.

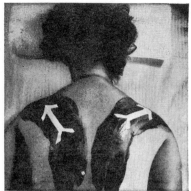

Figure 48
Middle and lower
trapezius, second division.°

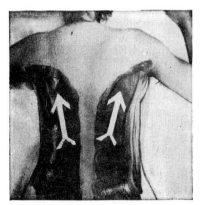

Figure 49
Latissimus dorsi,
third division.

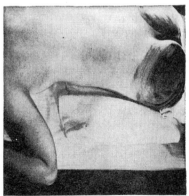

Figure 50
Gluteals, fourth division.

° The second division is not discussed in Miss McMillan's text, but is shown
in the illustration on page 27.

The glutei is the last division of the back. Here heavier pressure should be exerted on account of the density of fascia in this region. The operator, starting with one hand on each side of the buttocks, strokes from the apex of the sacrum over the whole of the gluteal muscles, coming back without pressure to the starting-point. When each division of the back has been effleuraged, it is well to cover the whole surface with long, firm, even strokes from the sacrum to the nape of the neck.

The back is divided in the same way for petrissage as for effleurage. Each section in turn is petrissaged by a pressure of muscles against the ribs, or, in the lumbar region, upon the abdominal wall. (sic) These muscles cannot be picked up as those in the limbs. The whole of the palmar surface of the hand is brought into play, but not in a molding manner as for the limbs, because the contour of the surface is flat instead of rounded.

The glutei muscles and fascia, being dense, require a much deeper kneading than those in any other region. The kneading movement over the glutei is similar to that in kneading dough. . . . After effleurage, petrissage, and tapotement of the first and second divisions of the back are completed, those parts are covered to protect them. The third and fourth divisions receive the same treatment, except that the glutei region, being more dense, gets beating instead of hacking. The cover is now entirely removed and the final procedure of effleurage is enacted, four to six strokes being administered, and each stroke extending the whole distance from the sacrum to the acromion. Tapotement in the form of brisk tapping for its stimulating effect, or light rhythmical hacking for its sedative effect, is used, according to the needs of the individual patient. Cupping the muscles, the hands being used alternately and making longitudinal sweeps each side of the spinal column, contributes the final procedure for the back.°

Summary

Mary McMillan's influence has been spread throughout the United States, Manila, China, and Europe. Her dynamic personality carried her to far parts of the world and wherever she went people could not help but feel her progressive influence. Through the army

° *Ibid.*, pp. 26–29, 33–34, 70.

training schools her techniques concerning positioning of the patient, maintaining contact on the return stroke, stroking off the whole area, and alternate-hand effleurage and petrissage became an integral part of massage in the United States.

18

James B. Mennell

Mennell says very little about the exact technique of massage except to describe the various strokes. He classifies these as: stroking, divided into superficial stroking and deep effleurage; and compression movements, divided into kneading, frictions, pressures, and petrissage. His terminology differs from common usage. He refers to friction as *frictions*, and divides petrissage into *kneading* and *petrissage*, the kneading referring to the circular, two-hand type of petrissage which is similar to Miss McMillan's two-hand petrissage.

Most of the emphasis in his book is placed on a slow and even rhythm, a gentle and light pressure, and a longer term of instruction for the masseur. A great deal of space is devoted to the physiological effects accomplished by massage rather than on the actual technique.

It is of maximum importance in massaging a given part to begin away from the part which is injured or diseased and work gradually toward it.

In reference to the patient's relaxation, Mennell states that:

The resistance offered by muscular contraction in the part under treatment to deep stroking is so great as to render it practically useless. As the first essential is to ensure that the whole part is in a state of perfect relaxation, careful attention must be given to the posture, not only of the part under treatment, but of the patient's whole body. If necessary, relaxation must be procured by preliminary superficial stroking. If the muscles are relaxed, they offer to the movement no more resistance than so much fluid, and therefore it is obvious that any pressure, exerted on the sur-

152

face, will be transmitted freely to all the structures under the hand. A pressure of 10 mm. of mercury will suffice to attain any objective desired by the use of the movement, except perhaps the mechanical emptying of a dilated lymphatic. A little practice, combined with a skill that is born only of a delicate sense of touch, will show how very light may be the pressure which will suffice to compress any structure to its full extent, and therefore, incidentally, to empty the veins and lymphatic spaces. Also there is no call for great rapidity of movement. The flow of blood in the veins is slow, and of the lymph in its channels still slower. There is no object in performing a movement to empty a vein if sufficient time has not elapsed for blood to flow into it, since the last movement ceased. Moreover, a heavy pressure, a very rapid movement, or even a jarring contact may convey to the patient the fear of a possible chance of injury, be the fear conscious or subconscious. A protective reflex may then be excited, the muscle may contract, and so the one condition under which we can perform our work to the greatest advantage is sacrificed. . . .

Unless contra-indications exist, we may take it for granted that deep stroking should commence over the proximal segment of a limb before we attack the distal, so as to ensure the "removal of the cork from the bottle".*

Regarding the patient's position, Mennell points out that the patient should be generally comfortable, with the head supported, abdominals and thigh muscles relaxed, and the feet supported. The therapist should maintain a stance which is in general comfortable, with no strain on the back muscles or knees. Her position should be such that she can reach the whole limb and support it properly.

Mennell's Techniques

Superficial stroking
Since superficial stroking is a distinctive part of Mennell's massage techniques, its description is here included in its entirety.

Though it is possible to trace a reflex response to most of the movements of massage, this is the only movement which aims at securing no other effect.

* Mennell, *op. cit.*, pp. 28–29.

The essentials to remember in using this treatment are that our movements must be slow, gentle, and rhythmical and yet they must be given with what one can only describe as a confident touch; there must be no doubt, hesitancy or irregularity about it.

The slowness is important, as without it the other two essentials are impossible. If the stroke is to pass from hand to shoulder, some fifteen movements a minute will suffice. Moreover, the movement of the masseur's hand throughout must be continuous and even, not only while the hand is in contact with the part, but also during the return through the air, when there must be no contact. Occasionally we hear it stated that loss of contact between the hand and the part is conducive to a chilling of the patient. This can only be due to inefficient performance, when the movement may convey a "creepy" sensation. This is usually the outcome of timidity, or of lack of training and practice.

The call for gentleness is obvious, as we are avowedly attempting to secure no mechanical effect. The firmness of the pressure should be sufficient only to ensure that the patient is actually conscious of the passage of the hand throughout the entire movement. Thus there should be no question of the patient being able to detect the passage of the hand over a certain point during one movement, while being unable to note it during subsequent movements. Otherwise the sensation conveyed by one movement cannot be identical with that conveyed by each subsequent movement. Firmness is essential, but only the lightest possible pressure.

The need for rhythm can be readily understood, as without it the nature of the stimulus will be uneven, and the reaction also will thereby be rendered uneven.

There should be no sensation of jarring at the beginning or end of the stroke, and the time that elapses between the end of one stroke and the commencement of the next must be identical throughout the whole of the treatment. To attain all these requisites it is essential to develop a "swing," and the portion of the "swing" which takes place while the hand is not in contact with the limb is as important as that during which hand and skin are in contact. Throughout the treatment the masseur's hand must remain supple, with all muscles relaxed, so that it may mould itself naturally to the contour of the limb, thus ensuring greater perfection of contact, and bringing as wide an area as possible under treatment. . . . If we wish to secure nothing but a reflex response to our movement, it may safely be left to the patient to decide the direction. If movement in one direction is more pleasing (*i.e.*, more sedative) than another, there can be no objection to using it, even though the movement be centrifugal.

Surface stroking "against the grain" of a hairy limb may be devoid of comfort, and, if so, it cannot be expected to call forth a beneficent reflex. It can only annoy. Shaving the part might be expected to help: it does not, and the process is not recommended save in the rarest of cases.

But whatever may be the direction chosen, one rule must be strictly obeyed, namely, that the stroking is performed in the one direction only. Thus, if we are stroking the back of a patient suffering from insomnia, our stroke should be from cervical or thoracic region downwards, or to the cervical or thoracic region upwards, never from sacrum to thoracic region and then out over the shoulder with a downward tendency at the end. In the same way, if a leg is being stroked upwards, the utmost care must be taken not to allow the hand to come into contact with any part of the limb during the return; otherwise the stimulus will be broken and the reaction thereby rendered imperfect. This is in direct opposition to the advice of a former writer to "feather your oars" when using stroking movements. By this he meant that heavy centripetal stroking should be followed by light centrifugal stroking. . . .

. . . The most common mistake is to scratch the patient with the pads of the fingers towards the end of each stroke. The second common error is to ignore the necessity for controlling the return of the hand through the air, and so to make this part of the movement less rhythmical than the stroking itself. A third main fault in technique is to ignore the necessity of selecting one definite direction for the movement, and, once having made the selection, of keeping to it. Another point, and one that is often overlooked, is that not only the hand, but every joint in the limb must be perfectly relaxed and perfectly supple.[*]

Deep effleurage

Mennell believes that this movement may be deep without being forcible, in any sense of the word. It is essential to ensure perfect relaxation (if necessary this can be acquired through superficial stroking). A pressure of 10 mm of mercury will suffice to obtain any objective desired by the use of the movement, except perhaps the mechanical emptying of a dilated lymphatic. Since the flow of blood and lymph is slow, this stroke should not be rapidly executed (Mennell, pp. 27–28).

[*] *Ibid.,* pp. 24–27.

Others

Aside from using *both hands simultaneously,* or *one hand at a time* as the occasion demands, Mennell does not use any other effleurage strokes.

Mennell distinguishes between kneading and petrissage, therefore, his description of both will be included here.

Kneading

This is performed with the two hands placed on opposite sides of the limb, the whole of the palmar surface being in contact with the part. Gentle pressure is then exerted and a circular movement performed, the hands usually working in an opposite direction. Pressure is so regulated that it is not even throughout the movement, but should be greatest while the hand is engaged with the lowest part of the circumference of the circle, and least when at the opposite pole. This is effected by imparting a slight rotation to the wrist, the hand being more supinated below than above. The movement commences over the proximal portion of the limb; the pressure is then reapplied at the next most distal part and the movement repeated (Mennell, p. 31).

Petrissage

The movement consists of grasping the muscle-mass between the fingers and thumbs of both hands and raising it away from the subjacent tissues. The tissues grasped are then compressed alternately between the thumb of one hand and the fingers of the other. The hands are made to slide away gently over the surface, until the whole region has been manipulated. Care should be taken to avoid an all-too-common error in technique: dragging the fingers over the surface. Instead of merely exerting an intermittent pressure, the grip should be soft and the whole hand relaxed (Fig. 51). Sometimes when the muscular tissue is sufficiently bulky, each picking-up movement is made to alternate with a kneading movement.

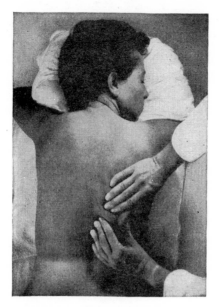

Figure 51
Mennell's petrissage on the back.

A third method, applicable chiefly to the calf, is performed by picking up the muscle in one or both hands and carrying it from side to side with an inclination to upward movement at the same time. The result is an almost semicircular movement. . . . Any movement that calls forth a protective contraction can only defeat our aims, and should be regarded as an error in technique.[*]

Friction

Regarding friction Mennell says:

In using frictions the object in view is to press deeply on the part under treatment and then to move the hand in a more or less circular direction. Any part of the hand may be used, but that generally employed is the tips of the fingers, or tip or ball of the thumb. . . .

[*] *Ibid.*, p. 39.

Friction directed transversely to the long axis of muscle fibers will often aid in securing relaxation.°

Although he says that any part of the hand may be used, he recommends the use of the *tips of the fingers and the ball of the thumb.*

Mennell's use of the term "frictions" instead of "friction" should be noted since he feels quite strongly that all massage is in a sense "friction," and therefore attempts to distinguish the terms by using this terminology.

Tapotement

Mennell describes tapotement under the title of "percussion movements."

Hacking. This may be performed with the ulnar border of the little finger, either alone or supplemented in turn by the other fingers—the result being a series of soft blows, the first from the little finger direct, the others from each successive finger in turn transmitted through the finger or fingers that have already delivered their tap. Sometimes the little finger is curled up in the palm of the hand, and only the middle fingers are used. If a more vigorous action is deemed necessary, the ulnar surface of the whole hand may be used with all the fingers kept close together and partially flexed but not rigid. The tips or palmar surfaces of the three middle fingers can be used. . . .

Clapping. The hands are so held that the fingers and palm form a concave arch, and in this position they are brought sharply into contact with the body. The result is a rather deep-toned clapping sound. . . .

Beating. This is the most vigorous form of percussion massage. The fist is half closed, and either the ulnar or the palmar surface is used for beating the surface of the body. If no force is put into the movement, it may be used over bony areas such as the sacrum and over areas well covered by muscle, such as the gluteal region. As our only hope from its use in these regions is to secure a reflex action it should be performed lightly.†

° *Ibid.*, pp. 33–34.

† *Ibid.*, pp. 40–41.

Vibration

Regarding vibration Mennell says:

> . . . hand vibration is a poor substitute for many of the mechanical vibrators on the market. . . . It is true that a few—a very few—masseurs have been able to develop a technique of administering vibration with their hands to such a degree of proficiency that manual treatment is preferable to that derived from apparatus.°

Summary

Mennell's theory of "uncorking the bottle" by massaging the proximal aspect of the limb before the distal is now being practiced by most therapists. As a rule they are following his principle of adapting the treatment to the individual patient's needs rather than treating by any specific routine concerning number of strokes or length of treatment. His influence has been widely felt throughout the United States. We must not forget his constant emphasis on the gentle approach, beginning away from the sensitive part and working slowly toward it. His use of massage, combined with careful relaxing passive movement, should always be kept in mind.

° *Ibid.*, p. 44.

19

James Cyriax

Cyriax feels that the most potent form of massage is deep friction. By this means, and by this means alone, massage can reach to structures far below the surface of the body. If damage is to be avoided the physical therapist must know how to give it and exactly where to give it. Deep friction can be given with advantage only to the site of the lesion, which may or may not be within the painful area outlined by the patient. It is only when a deeply situated soft structure has to have mobility restored that penetrating massage should be given.

In his text, *Treatment by Manipulation and Massage,* Cyriax sets forth the following beliefs.*

The principle governing the treatment of muscles during the acute or chronic stage is the same. The endeavour must be to prevent the continued adherence of unwanted young fibrous tissue in recent cases, or to rupture adherent scar-tissue in long-standing cases. To stretch out a muscle does not widen the distance between its fibers; on the contrary, during stretching they lie more closely. Whereas, then, for the rupture of adherent scars about a joint mobilization is required, interfibrillary adhesions in muscle can be broken, not by stretching, but by forcibly broadening the muscle out. Particularly is this true of the fibres of attachment of muscle into bone, where the rupture of adhesions is possible only by means of friction or subcutaneous division. Thus, *deep transverse frictions restore mobility to muscle in the same way as mobilization frees*

* James Cyriax: *Treatment by Manipulation and Massage.* Paul B. Hoeber, Inc., New York (Published in England under the title *Orthopaedic Medicine, Volume II: Treatment by Manipulation and Massage* by Cassell and Company Ltd., London) 1959.

a joint. Indeed, *the action of deep transverse frictions may be summed up as affording a mobilization such as passive stretching or active exercise cannot achieve.*

After the friction has restored a full range of painless broadening to the muscle belly, this added mobility must be maintained. To this end, the patient must perform a series of active contractions with the joint placed in the position that fully relaxes the affected muscle, *i.e.*, the position that allows the greatest broadening. Strong resisted movements should be avoided until the scar has consolidated itself otherwise, started too soon, they tend to open the healing breach again. Athletes in particular must not return to full sport too early.

Deep Massage in Treatment of Ligaments

In recent cases, after any oedema that may be present has been removed by effleurage, the site of the minor tear in the ligament should receive some minutes friction. The purpose is to disperse blood-clot or effusion here, to move the ligament to and fro over subjacent bone in imitation of its normal behavior (thus maintaining its mobility) and to numb it enough to facilitate movement afterwards. The least strength of friction that achieves these results is called for. Passive then active movements follow. After a short time, the effleurage becomes less necessary and more attention is devoted to the friction and to exercising the injured limb under supervision. In the case of the lower limb instruction in gait follows.

In chronic cases deep friction is given to fibrous structures such as ligaments in preparation for mobilization. In such cases the friction thins out the scar-tissue by which the fibrous structure is held abnormally adherent, and so numbs it that mobilization becomes possible.

Deep Massage in Treatment of Tendons

In acute and chronic teno-synovitis the way deep massage acts appears somewhat different. On logical grounds it has been widely held that teno-synovitis, being as a rule the result of overuse, should not be treated by further friction. Nevertheless this is the very condition in which massage achieves some of its quickest and most brilliant results. The phenomenon of crepitus proves that roughening of the gliding surfaces occurs. The fact that slitting up the sheath of the tendon at open operation is immediately curative shows that it was the movement between the close-fitting sheath and the tendon that set up the pain. Hence it would appear that manual rolling of the tendon-sheath to and fro against the tendon serves to smooth the gliding surfaces off again. While the causative trauma was longitudinal friction the curative is transverse.

In those tendons that lack a sheath the way deep massage acts is not so clear. After minor teno-periosteal tears the movement imparted by the massage, when successful, presumably breaks up scarring at the insertion of tendon into bone. When the substance of a tendon such as the supraspinatus is affected, it is difficult to understand exactly what the massage can do unless it is assumed that scar-tissue lies here and is capable of mobilization manually. Since no sheath exists, there is no reason to suppose that some slight roughening of the surface of the tendon would cause symptoms. Nevertheless, deep friction provides the only method known to me of bringing lasting relief quickly in such cases, apart from recent experience with hydrocortisone.*

Technique of Deep Friction

When massage is to be given to muscle, tendon, ligament or joint-capsule, two principles must be observed. They are that the massage must be given (*a*) to the right spot, and (*b*) in the most effective way. Clearly, only the place whence a pain springs requires treatment, but the referred pain so often present in the conditions sent to a Physiotherapy Department creates immediate difficulty; for the site of the pain and even of the tenderness do not then correspond with the site of the lesion. Since deep massage applies therapeutic movement only locally, it is by no means enough merely to apply friction somewhere close to a lesion. To give massage to a normal structure only a fraction of an inch away from the correct spot, is, in my view, quite valueless. There are many conditions unsuited to treatment by deep massage; these should not receive it. There exist other disorders calling for friction; this must then be given to the exact spot whence the pain originates, but it must be remembered that this does not necessarily lie within the area in which the patient *feels* the pain.

Once agreement has been reached on the truism that the actual site of the lesion alone requires treatment, the question naturally arises of how a penetrating effect is best imparted to massage. The principles are:

1. The right spot must be found.

The identification of the precise spot where the physiotherapist must apply her finger depends entirely on knowledge of anatomy. For example, at the shoulder massage is often given to a stated part of a stated structure and no question arises of asking the patient if that spot is tender or not; at other sites the diagnostic movements may have singled out the tissue at fault, search for tenderness *along that structure* picking out the exact site of the lesion.

* *Ibid.*, pp. 15–16.

I consider it part of the physiotherapist's duty, when asked to give massage to a named structure, to judge which part of that structure is affected and to give treatment directly to that spot only. Adequate time must be spent in identifying the exact point where she shall apply her finger.

2. The physiotherapist's fingers and the patient's skin must move as one.

Should movement take place between the patient's skin and the physiotherapist's fingers, then the friction is expended on the patient's skin. When penetration is required, this can be secured only by rubbing the patient's skin and subcutaneous fascia against his muscle, ligament or tendon. The whole art of giving deep friction without damaging the patient's skin depends on mastery of this technique. Vigorous friction between the physiotherapist's finger and the patient's skin soon raises a blister. When, on the other hand, the skin and superficial tissues are drawn to and fro over the area to be treated, they stand the strain perfectly well. Some transient redness of the skin usually follows, but no more. Occasionally, in fat patients, a little subcutaneous bruising may appear a day or two after the massage; rarely a nodule may form in the adipose layer. The patient is usually quite unconscious of either, and both soon disappear. Sometimes it may be advisable to alter the area of skin receiving pressure from time to time during one session. The finger may be applied to the lesion after the skin has been drawn to one or other side. When the choice has to be made, it is always preferable to be sure of reaching the right spot than to spare the patient some hours' soreness of his skin. The doctor must back the physiotherapist up should a patient complain; he has only to point out that deep massage to a tender point cannot be painless for the patient to understand the position.

3. The friction must be given *across* the fibers composing the affected structure.

Striated structures must receive massage given transversely. It is only thus that each fibre is drawn away from its fellow and mobility restored to muscle; it is thus that a ligament is made to reproduce its normal movement over bone; and it is thus that the surface of a tendon may be smoothed off. The thicker and stronger the structure, the more must friction be given to it strictly across the grain.

4. The friction must be given with sufficient sweep.

The amplitude of the to-and-fro movement of the physiotherapist's fingers must be great enough to ensure that the frictional element is paramount. Only thus can effective separation of each fibre from its fellow be secured. The limiting factors are only the size of the area requiring treatment and the elasticity of the overlying skin. In this connexion it is unfortunate that students are often taught to impart deep friction by a circular movement of the thumbs. When this method is used for deeply situated lesions no physiotherapist—however strong her hands—can avoid giving what amounts to pressure without enough friction. This should be avoided as it is painful and seldom curative.

It is a grave fault when, in giving massage, pressure replaces, instead of augments, friction. Thus, while it is true that adequate massage to an inflamed, and therefore tender, spot is bound to be painful, the fact that massage is painful is no guarantee that it is correctly given. *Unless the friction is given with a sufficient transverse sweep its curative value is largely lost.*

5. The friction must reach deeply enough.

The vigour with which deep massage is given is proportional to the toughness and distance from the surface of the tissue at fault. When, for example, the thick tendons at the shoulder require treatment, the limiting factor is the physiotherapist's strength. She cannot rub hard enough to do harm; her difficulty is to rub hard enough to do good.

The frictional element in deep massage is always paramount; pressure augments, but must never replace, friction. If this essential point is neglected a most painful treatment results which has no curative value. Hence, while proper massage to a tender area is bound to hurt, the mere fact of hurting affords no proof that the technique is correct. Indeed, deep friction, skilfully given, hurts less than when given by a novice. During each session physiotherapists unaccustomed to this sort of work do better to give a friction that really reaches the lesion for a few minutes at a time, pausing between whiles, than to rub gently, and hence in vain, for a longer period.

6. The patient must adopt a suitable position.

A position must be adopted that ensures the requisite degree of tension on, or relaxation of, the tissue to be treated. Some structures, notably the tendons about the shoulder, lie out of reach of a physiotherapist's finger unless the patient is first put into the position dictated by anatomical considerations.

7. Muscles must be kept relaxed while being given friction.

When, as is common, the substance of a muscle rather than its surface is affected, the massage must penetrate deeply. Hence the patient must keep his muscle relaxed throughout the administration of the massage. Since his instinct is to steel himself against the discomfort of the friction by contracting his muscle, he has to learn to avoid this reaction. Moreover, he must be placed in a position in which the part controlled by that muscle lies limply. . . .

8. Tendons with a sheath must be kept taut while being given friction.
In teno-synovitis the roughening is confined to the outer surface of the tendon and the inner surface of its sheath. The friction is intended to smooth off the two gliding surfaces. To this end the tendon must be stretched so that it forms an immobile basis against which to move the sheath. Should the tendon remain lax, it and its sheath are rolled against adjacent structures and little good results.°

If much deep friction is to be given in the course of a day, it is essential to use the hands alternately, and to use now the fingers, now the thumb, for affecting the same place. Full ambidexterity is most useful. When part of a limb is to be treated, the physiotherapist's hand is as a rule best used in a grasping position.

The ability to continue friction for a considerable time is increased by sharing the work out among different muscles of the physiotherapist's limb. For example, if the finger or thumb is held firmly against the structure to be treated, and the friction is induced by a wrist, elbow, shoulder or trunk movement, two sets of muscles are in action and more power is achieved for less effort. No matter how strong the physiotherapist, she cannot give effective friction by alternate flexion and extension movements of the fingers or thumb. *The whole hand must move.* Massage must not be given with the fingers hyperextended, for the capsules of the interphalangeal joints soon become painfully strained. The fingers should be kept slightly flexed during heavy massage, and the necessary strength of the forearm muscles acquired. It should not be necessary to add that when the hand is used in this position the finger-nails must be kept quite short.

Suitable positions of the physiotherapist's hands
There are four main ways in which a physiotherapist may use her hand to the best advantage. They are:

1. The Index crossed over the Middle Finger
(Occasionally one thumb may be used instead of the crossed fingers.) This technique is well suited to linear areas, such as the attachment of a ribbon of tissue to bone: for example, the occipital insertion of the trapezeus or the fibular origin of the lateral ligament of the ankle. This is also the best way to affect a supraspinous ligament or the coronary liga-

° *Ibid.,* pp. 19–22.

ment at the knee. This position of the fingers is also required when massage is given to a structure ensconced between two bones, *e.g.* the tendon of the tibialis posterior. One finger should be pressed on to the lesion and the friction imparted by rolling the finger to and fro over it. This movement is set up by alternating rotation of the forearm.

2. *The Middle Finger crossed over Index*

When a structure forming part of a limb is to be treated, the physiotherapist naturally grasps the limb, thus using her thumb for counter-pressure. The fact of curving the fingers means that the index no longer reaches to the distal phalanx of the middle finger; hence the tip of the middle finger should reinforce the index on the nail.

3. *Two Finger-tips*

Depending on how the fibres of the structure to be massaged run in relation to the physiotherapist's hand, the index and middle finger-tips, or the middle and ring finger-tips, should be used. The belly of any flat muscle can be suitably dealt with in this way.

4. *The Opposed Fingers and Thumb*

This is the pinching position. The physiotherapist, having grasped the structure, applies friction by pulling her hand towards herself. The tendons at the shoulder, the medial ligament at the knee, the biceps brachii muscle, and the tendo Achillis provide instances of this usage.[*]

Summary

This outline of Cyriax's basic principles of massage explains his important contribution to contemporary massage technique. His book does a magnificent illustrative job of demonstrating specific application of these techniques to various areas of the body for specific conditions. It is the belief of this author that his text should be a part of every massage library.

[*] *Ibid.*, pp. 24–25.

20

An Introduction to Bindegewebsmassage

This brief discussion of a technique which is being used in Germany and, to some extent, throughout Europe, is *deliberately lacking in detail*. Although specific instructions have been translated into English they will not be included here until further research has indicated exactly what effects this type of treatment has on the entire organism. Little has been done to prove whether or not the effects can be controlled.

Since this technique is so specific, it would not be wise to include detailed instructions here without assurance that the therapist using this approach has also had demonstrations and supervised practice.

Elisabeth Dicke claims that the effects of this type of massage could bring about harmony in the autonomic nervous system, influence regulatory dysfunction based on vegetational autonomic disturbances, stimulate in cases of vegetational dysfunction, release spasm by influencing vascular regulation, and influence hyperergic reactions in allergic patients.

Frau Dicke observed changes of tension of the connective tissue in segments that correlated (according to Head and MacKenzie) to diseased organs of the viscera. She could palpate these changes as swellings, contractions, or depressions.

The basic treatment starts in the caudal area and continues, ascending gradually toward the cranium in three sequences. Treatment always starts from the median line of the spinal cord and goes from the radicular segments to the involved peripheral segments.

The finger tips of the middle and fourth fingers pass through the superficial tissues with a light pull and lift, producing a specific stimulus to the connective tissue. The skin is moved against its bony or muscular base. By working along the bony edges of the skeleton, muscle insertions, fascia, and tendons, and working from superficial tissues to deeper layers, Frau Dicke believes that specific reflex effects can be brought about. The technique should be carried out precisely in accordance with the anatomical structure of the body.

If possible the patient is placed in a sitting position, or, if necessary the treatment can be given with the patient lying down. The treatment usually takes about thirty minutes, following which the patient should rest from thirty minutes to an hour. These treatments are given in series of about twelve to eighteen, and, depending on the tolerance of the patient, work gradually upward from day to day unless only the lower part of the body is involved.

Summary

Interest in massage techniques took this author to Germany to study Bindegewebsmassage at the Elisabeth Dicke School. There seems little doubt that this technique can produce *some* of the reflex effects which it claims are possible. The book, *Massage, Manipulation and Traction,* edited by Sidney Licht (published by Elizabeth Licht, New York, 1960) covers Bindegewebsmassage more thoroughly. However, it is not the feeling of this author that these techniques should be used until more research has been done in this field.

Recommended Readings for Part III

Cyriax, James: *Treatment by Manipulation and Deep Massage,* 6th ed. Paul B. Hoeber, New York (Published in England under the title *Orthopaedic Medicine, Volume II: Treatment by Manipulation and Massage* by Cassell and Company, Ltd., London) 1959.

Dicke, Elisabeth: *Meine Bindegewebsmassage.* Hippokrates-Verlag, Stuttgart, 1956, pp. 7–15.

Ebner, M.: "Peripheral Circulatory Disturbances: Treatment by Massage of Connective Tissue Reflex Zones," *Brit. J. Phys. Med.,* Vol. 19, (Aug.) 1956, pp. 176–80.

Hoffa, Albert J.: *Technik der Massage,* 3rd ed. Ferdinand Enke, Stuttgart, 1900.

McMillan, Mary: *Massage and Therapeutic Exercise,* 3rd ed. W. B. Saunders Co., 1932.

Mennell, James B.: *Physical Treatment by Movement, Manipulation, and Massage,* 5th ed. The Blakiston Co., Philadelphia, J. and A. Churchill, Ltd., London, 1945.

This book has described massage as it is being done in America today. It varies little from techniques used over the last hundred years in Europe or America. It should. Massage as we are doing it is pragmatically useful. However, just as recent research in neuromuscular facilitation has radically changed methods of therapeutic exercise, similar study, particularly into the reflex effects of massage, could necessitate equally interesting changes in massage techniques.

Appendix

Review Questions

These questions are designed to help the student evaluate the amount of knowledge he has been able to assimilate.

1. Define massage.
2. Give three purposes each for massage being used (a) in nursing, (b) in physical education, and (c) in physical therapy.
3. On what basis would you judge treatment time for various patients?
4. Outline the important factors of personal appearance and cleanliness.
5. Why are postural considerations important to the therapist?
6. Name ten ways to assure comfort for the patient.
7. Name four fundamental facts pertaining to proper positioning of patients.
8. Outline the basic principles for draping a patient.
9. List the deciding factors in choice of lubricant.
10. Name six lubricants and tell when you might use each.
11. Describe effleurage.
12. Diagram draping and positioning for massage of the back.
13. When lying prone what consideration should be given to the position of the arms?
14. Describe all variations of effleurage.
15. Define the usefulness of petrissage.
16. List ten desirable qualities of personality of the therapist.
17. Describe draping of the lower extremity, face-lying.

18. Briefly explain the place each name has in the history of massage and rearrange the names chronologically:
    a. Ambroise Paré
    b. Hartvig Nissen
    c. Albert Hoffa
    d. J. M. M. Lucas-Championnière
    e. Mary McMillan
    f. Hwang-Ti
    g. Hippocrates
    h. Per Henrik Ling
    i. Gertrude Beard
    j. Homer
    k. James B. Mennell
    l. Elisabeth Dicke
    m. Sir William Bennett
19. How can you judge how much lubricant to use?
20. How does Storm's technique vary from the usual type of friction?
21. Would you ever give massage for skin nutrition only?
22. What is the effect of massage on sensory nerve endings?
23. How would you know when it was safe to massage scar tissue following burns?
24. What would massage do to effect normal function of the skin?
25. What is meant by reflex effects?
26. List the mechanical effects of massage.
27. Why should massage be done slowly if the objective is to assist the lymphatic flow?
28. Why is it important to rid the muscle of stagnant by-products of fatigue?
29. Explain how muscles normally maintain a metabolic balance.
30. Why is massage useful following overactivity?
31. Describe the metabolic picture following underactivity.
32. What is meant by venostasis?

33. Name three instances when you would *not* massage situations showing venostasis.
34. Name and explain four causes of edema.
35. Why does swelling occur in dependent limbs when normal activity has been limited?
36. Will massage be useful in eliminating edema in limbs suffering from extreme activity?
37. Why is massage not recommended in cases where edema is the result of recent injury?
38. Why is research in massage so difficult?
39. Will massage reduce obesity?
40. Of what use is massage following peripheral nerve injuries?
41. Does massage effect total blood flow?
42. Is massage more effective than electrical stimulation or passive exercise in increasing the flow of lymph?
43. Can massage ever adequately substitute for active exercise?
44. Describe massage as done by Cyriax.

Summary Chart of Comparative Techniques

The following summary chart shows the results of a questionnaire used to determine the amount of use generally given to the various massage techniques. Twenty-five graduate therapists were interviewed from fifteen different schools. These schools were: D.T. Watson School of Physical Therapy (Leetsdale, Pennsylvania); Children's Hospital (Los Angeles, California); Harvard University, Medical School, Courses for Graduates (Boston, Massachusetts); University of Southern California (Los Angeles, California); Mayo Clinic (Rochester, Minnesota); University of Minnesota (Minneapolis, Minnesota); Northwestern University, Medical School (Chicago, Illinois); New York University, School of Education (New York City); Stanford University (Stanford, California); University of Wisconsin, Medical School (Madison, Wisconsin); Reed College * (Portland, Oregon); Fitzsimmons General Hospital * (Denver, Colorado); O'Reilly General Hospital * (Springfield, Missouri); Walter Reed General Hospital * (Washington, D.C.); and The Institute of Southern Sweden (Stockholm, Sweden).

In order to prevent any one school from influencing the results, not more than three from each school were interviewed. In some instances, where the therapist was teaching in one school but a graduate of another, it was considered that the information gathered was representative of the school in which she was now teaching.

* Army Training Schools.

QUESTION	HOFFA	McMILLAN
1. Are there any exceptions to following the venous flow?	The only exception is in the massage of the back, where the stroke may go in either direction.	No exceptions are made.
2. What do you consider adequate treatment time for the back, a limb, and total body?	Six to ten minutes is used for back or limb and fifteen minutes for whole body.	Ten to fifteen minutes is recommended for beginners to use for the back or limb and not more than fifty minutes for a general massage.
3. What do you prefer as a medium?	Anything to make the part pliable can be used.	Dry rubbing is preferred but for certain pathologies oil, cocoa butter or lanolin is suggested.
4. Do you massage by muscle groups or is massage done by other anatomical divisions of the body?	All massage is done by dividing the body into various muscle groups.	Some areas are divided by muscle groups and others, such as the back, are described, using other anatomical landmarks.

The first column of the chart gives the questions asked; the second, third, and fourth columns explain, in brief, the methods of Hoffa, Miss McMillan, and Minnell; and the last column gives the conclusions arrived at from the questionnaire results.

MENNELL	CONCLUSIONS FROM QUESTIONNAIRE RESULTS
Exceptions include superficial stroking and following the principle of beginning away from the injured area.	The trend seems to be progressively toward making exceptions to following the venous flow as Mennell does.
Treatment time must depend on the pathology and reaction of the patient. No time can be suggested.	Treatment time must be adjustable to the pathology and reactions of the patient, but average between ten to twenty minutes for back or limb and up to forty-five for the whole body, which is more than Hoffa recommends and similar to McMillan's suggested time.
Mennell's prescription combines oil of Bergamot and French chalk.	Except in cases where pathology demands one or the other, choice of medium is up to the therapist, as Hoffa suggests.
Only the fact that one begins away from the injured part and works toward it, is mentioned as to how the area is covered.	The majority of therapists still divide the body into specific muscle groups for massage as Hoffa does.

QUESTION	HOFFA	McMILLAN
5. Is the most proximal part of the limb massaged before the distal?	Every description of a part to be massaged progresses from the distal aspect of the limb to the proximal.	Descriptions progress from the distal aspect of the limb to the proximal.
6. Is the whole extremity or back effleuraged before petrissage is begun?	Each muscle or muscle group is given effleurage and petrissage before the next group is begun.	Massage of the leg is done by giving effleurage to the whole lower leg and then petrissage.
7. Is the patient always placed in a recumbent position?	The only place that the patient is in a recumbent position is in massage of the back, and even here the patient may be in a seated position.	The patient is always in a recumbent position unless pathology is such that this position cannot be held comfortably.
8. Which parts are usually supported, (1) in a back-lying position, and (2) in a face-lying position?	(1) No back-lying position is described. (2) No mention of support is made with reference to the face-lying position.	(1) A rolled towel is placed under the knee. (2) A small pillow is placed under the abdomen.

MENNELL	CONCLUSIONS FROM QUESTIONNAIRE RESULTS
The proximal aspect of a limb should always be massaged before the more distal.	The practice of massaging the most proximal aspect of a limb before the distal as Mennell recommends is now being widely used.
No definite routine in this respect is stated.	Most therapists are still following the technique of massaging each muscle or muscle group with effleurage and petrissage before going to the next group as Hoffa does, rather than effleuraging a whole part and then giving it petrissage.
The patient is preferred in a recumbent position, but each patient must be considered individually. Thus sitting, or even standing positions may be used if necessary.	Most massage to the upper extremity is done with the patient in a seated position. The tendency seems to be that of making exceptions to the recumbent position as Mennell does.
(1) Support is placed under the knee. (2) The body is supported in slight hyperextension for back massage, with one pillow under the legs and another under the chest.	(1) Knees are supported in the back-lying position as by McMillan and Mennell. (2) Most therapists follow the technique of McMillan and support the abdomen, and all but three support the ankles or have them over edge of the plinth.

QUESTION	HOFFA	McMILLAN
9. What arm position is preferred when the patient is face-lying?	The arms are "out horizontally."	Arms are shown in "T" position and also down at the sides.
10. In massage of the lower extremity is the patient usually turned from back-lying to face-lying?	The patient is turned to make the posterior thigh more accessible and is placed on the side to massage the tensor fascia lata.	The patient is not usually turned, but may be if pathological conditions are such that it seems best to do so.
11. Must the part being massaged always be in elevation?	It is believed that Hoffa prefers a neutral position.	All illustrations show the part in a neutral position.
12. Is emphasis placed on stance of the therapist?	No reference is made to stance.	No reference is made to stance.
13. Do you alternate sides of the table during massage of the back?	The therapist is instructed to move to the opposite side of the back when doing the other side.	No reference is made as to alternating sides of the table in massage of the back.

MENNELL	CONCLUSIONS FROM QUESTIONNAIRE RESULTS
Arms are folded over the head. (Chest is supported by a pillow which relieves weight on the arms.)	McMillan's two positions are the ones used the most ("T" and at the sides), but the patient's comfort and ability to relax is the primary guide for selection of arm position.
The patient is turned to make the posterior thigh more accessible.	McMillan's policy of not turning the patient unless pathology indicates its necessity seems to be followed.
Elevation is preferred whenever possible.	According to Hoffa and McMillan, the trend is still that of elevating the part for pathological conditions and treating it otherwise in a neutral position.
Mennell mentions the therapist should stand at the side of the table and not at the end. He should be comfortable with no strain on the back or knees.	Little emphasis other than good body mechanics is placed on stance by anyone.
Mennell does alternate sides of the table during a back massage.	McMillan and the majority of the therapists do not alternate sides of the table during massage of the back.

QUESTION	HOFFA	McMILLAN
14. Do you always massage in a standing position?	Most of the massage is done with the therapist seated, even in giving a massage to the back.	All illustrations show the therapist in a standing position.
15. Do you usually repeat a given stroke any particular number of times before progressing to a different stroke?	Hoffa refers to repeating a stroke "three or four" times but sets up no definite routine.	Suggestions for "three or four" strokes are included in descriptions. The number of strokes vary up to six and no set number is recommended.
16. Does return stroke always maintain contact?	It is believed that Hoffa does not maintain contact with his return stroke.	The hand should return to its original position without pressure but without losing contact with the part being massaged.
17. Do you ever "stroke off" a whole area, such as the back, the upper extremity, or the lower extremity?	No description of such a technique can be found in Hoffa's text.	The back is stroked off when each division has been effleuraged and on the forearm as a final stroke.

MENNELL	CONCLUSIONS FROM QUESTIONNAIRE RESULTS
It is advised that all massage be done in a standing position.	Whereas the therapists do not remain seated to the extent that Hoffa did, neither do they stand without exception. Hands and forearms are usually done with the therapist seated.
Mennell makes no reference to number of strokes to be given.	The trend seems away from grouping strokes by numbers as indicated by the lack of mention of such in Mennell's text and the fact that the majority of the therapists interviewed do not do so, except as a guide for beginners, which may have been all the basic texts meant it for (by the way it was mentioned).
The return stroke does not always maintain contact with the body, particularly with superficial stroking.	McMillan's technique of maintaining contact on the return stroke is being used by most of the therapists.
Mennell's "superficial stroking" is similar but of a superficial nature only.	McMillan's influence has been felt in that she and the majority of the therapists use this technique.

USE OF THE VARIOUS STROKES

QUESTION	HOFFA	McMILLAN
1. Which of the effleurage strokes are used?	Hoffa describes the use of: Light and deep stroking Knuckling Circular effleurage Thumb stroking Alternate-thumb stroking Simultaneous stroking.	McMillan describes the use of: Light and deep stroking Simultaneous stroking Alternate-hand stroking.
2. Which of the petrissage strokes are used?	Hoffa describes the use of petrissage which is: One-handed Two-handed (with flat hand for large flat surfaces and pick up where possible) Two-fingered.	McMillan describes the use of petrissage which is: One-handed Two-handed With alternate hands Finger and thumb For small areas Flat-handed on the back.

MENNELL	CONCLUSIONS FROM QUESTIONNAIRE RESULTS
Mennell describes the use of: Superficial stroking Deep effleurage Simultaneous stroking.	The majority of the therapists use an effleurage that is predominantly the same, light and deep stroking, and simultaneous stroking. Alternate-hand stroking which was mentioned by McMillan is widely used as well as one-hand-over-the-other for deeper pressure. Also of note is the tendency for the therapists to pick up Mennell's idea of superficial stroking, although they do not do it in the prescribed manner.
Mennell describes use of: Kneading (circular movements in opposite directions) Petrissage (raising muscle mass away from subjacent tissues) One-handed.	Hoffa's techniques for petrissage are predominantly in use; McMillan's two-hand petrissage and Mennell's are very similar and this stroke is used by some.

QUESTION	HOFFA	McMILLAN
3. Which of the friction strokes are used?	Hoffa describes the use of friction which uses: The thumb The index finger Both thumb and index finger.	McMillan describes the use of friction which uses: The thumb Two or three fingers The thenar eminence.
4. a. Is tapotement used routinely? b. Which of the tapotement strokes are used?	a. Tapotement is used routinely. b. Hacking is the only tapotement stroke that is described.	a. McMillan describes the use of tapotement routinely for a general massage. b. Tapotement strokes described are: Hacking Clapping Tapping Beating.
5. How is vibration used?	Hoffa does vibration either with the points of the fingers or with a flat hand but advises the use of a mechanical vibrator.	McMillan describes vibration as being done with one finger or several and also with the flat hand.

MENNELL	CONCLUSIONS FROM QUESTIONNAIRE RESULTS
Mennell describes friction which uses any part of the hand, but especially the tips of the fingers or the balls of the thumbs.	Use of the heel of the hand and one-over-the-other for pressure are not described by any of the basic texts, but are being used widely. Other techniques concerning friction are predominantly the same, except for the few therapists who combine friction and petrissage into a stroke which resembles both strokes.
a. Mennell describes the use of tapotement but does not use it routinely. b. He describes the use of: Hacking Clapping Beating.	a. Whereas Hoffa used tapotement routinely and McMillan described its use in a general massage, Mennell states that he does not use it routinely and the majority of the therapists use it for certain pathological conditions only. b. Use of the various strokes is fairly unified.
Mennell believes that the hand is a poor substitute for a mechanical vibrator.	Although described by all three of the basic texts, it is used very little.

QUESTION	HOFFA	McMILLAN
6. Which other strokes are used?	None.	The five fundamental procedures can form the basis for a large variety of manipulations.

MENNELL	CONCLUSIONS FROM QUESTIONNAIRE RESULTS
Mennell describes "shaking" in which the hand grasps the part giving quick firm vibrations which shake it from side to side. He also mentions a stroke which is similar to friction, but it is applied in a transverse plane to the muscle fibers.	Horizontal stroking for the low back is rather widely used although very few have a name for this stroke. Mennell's frictionlike stroke, which is done in a transverse plane, is used by some. Although used by only a few, Storm's technique for nodules has made some impression in this country.

Suggestions for Practical Testing

Students' applications of massage techniques are difficult to evaluate, and grades are often subjective. Students have the right to as accurate an evaluation as possible. The following chart is suggested as a means to a numerical evaluation on which a grade can be given. Apparent weaknesses can also be noted.

With this form the instructor can list an entire class on one page, making possible a comparison of all marks. There are twenty-four items to evaluate, each which can be given a maximum score of 4. This gives a numerical total of 96 and allows 4 points which can be subtracted or added under "remarks" for incidentals not listed among the other twenty-four. These could be such things as "leaning on the patient," or "dragging a towel or sleeve across the part to be treated."

In this way the instructor can justify the grade by showing a numerical mark. It also provides a written record which can be gone over with the student.

Some instructors may prefer a briefer form. On page 192 is a form which can be used for one student. This leaves more room for remarks than the one previously shown. It can also be evaluated numerically.

Practical Evaluation Sheet for Instructor's Use in Massage

TECHNIQUE OF STUDENT	Name of Student												
DRAPING													
POSITIONING													
EFFLEURAGE, RHYTHM													
" PRESSURE													
" PATTERN													
PETRISSAGE, RHYTHM													
" PRESSURE													
" PROGRESSION													
FRICTION, RHYTHM													
" PRESSURE													
" PATTERN													
TAPOTEMENT, RHYTHM													
" PRESSURE													
" PATTERN													
VIBRATION													
OTHER STROKES													
USE OF LUBRICANT													
POSTURE OF STUDENT													
CONDITION OF HANDS													
PERSONAL APPEARANCE													
KNOWLEDGE OF CASE													
ATTITUDE, POISE													
OVER-ALL APPROACH													
CLEAN UP													
REMARKS													
NUMERICAL TOTAL													
FINAL GRADE													

GRADING KEY
A—Excellent   4
B—Above Average   3   Remarks
C—Average   2
D—Below Average   1
F—Failing   0

Practical Evaluation Sheet for Instructor's Use in Massage

Student's Name _____

Statement of Problem or Case:

	GRADE	REMARKS
+10 POSITIONING		
+10 DRAPING		
+10 CHOICE AND USE OF LUBRICANT		
+20 ORGANIZATION OVER-ALL APPROACH		
+20 SKILL IN TECHNIQUE		
+10 TERMINATION DRESSING, ETC.		
+20 OVER-ALL IMPRESSION		
FINAL GRADE		

Bibliography

Alexander, R. S.: "The Physiology and Measurement of Peripheral Circulation," *Phys. Therapy Rev.*, Vol. 30, No. 11, (Nov.) 1950, pp. 452–61.

Bard, P.: *Medical Physiology.* C. V. Mosby Co., St. Louis, 1956.

Barker, R. C.; Wright, B. A.; and Gonick, Mollie R.: *Adjustment to Physical Handicap and Illness.* Social Science Research Council, New York, Bulletin No. 55, 1946.

Barron, D. J.: *Physiology of the Organs of Circulation of the Blood and Lymph, Sec. VI, Textbook of Physiology* (edited by J. F. Fulton). W. B. Saunders Co., Philadelphia, 1955.

Bauer, W. W.; Short, C. L.; and Bennett, G. A.: "Manner of Removal of Protein from Normal Joints," *J. Exp. Med.*, Vol. 57, No. 419, 1933.

Beard, Gertrude: "A History of Massage Technic," *Phys. Therapy Rev.*, Vol. 32, No. 12, (Dec.) 1952, pp. 613–14.

Best, C. H., and Taylor, N. B.: *The Living Body*, 4th ed. Holt, Rinehart and Winston, Inc., New York, 1958.

Beutner, R.; Calesmick, M. S.; Powell, E.; and Bortin, L.: "On the Absorption and Excretion of Methylsalicylate Administered by Inunction," *J. Lab. & Clin. Med.*, Vol. 14, No. 1655, (Nov.) 1951.

Blasko, J. J.: "Some Psychiatric Aspects in a Physical Therapy Program," *Phys. Therapy Rev.*, Vol. 31, No. 11, (Nov.) 1951, pp. 468–73.

Carrier, E. B.: "Determination of Plasma and Hemoglobin Volumes after Unit Hemorrhages under Controlled Experimental Conditions," *Ann. of Physiol.*, Vol. 61, No. 528, 1922.

193

Chor, H.; Cleveland, D.; Davenport, H. A.; Dolkart, R. A.; and Beard, G.: "Atrophy and Regeneration of the Gastrocnemius-Soleus Muscles," *J. A. M. A.*, Vol. 113, No. 1029, (Sept.) 1939.

Copestake, B. M. G.: *The Theory and Practice of Massage*, 4th ed. Paul B. Hoeber, Inc., New York, 1926.

Cyriax, J.: *Treatment by Manipulation and Deep Massage*, 6th ed. Paul B. Hoeber, Inc., New York, 1959.

Dicke, Elisabeth: *Meine Bindegewebsmassage*. Hippokrates-Verlag, Stuttgart, 1956.

Ebel, A., and Wisham, L.: "Effect of Massage on Muscle Temperature and Radiosodium Clearance," *Arch. Phys. Med.*, Vol. 33, No. 7, (July) 1952, pp. 399–405.

Ebner, M.: "Peripheral Circulatory Disturbances: Treatment by Massage of Connective Tissue Reflex Zones," *Brit. J. Phys. Med.*, Vol. 19, (Aug.) 1956, pp. 176–80.

Elkins, E. C.; Herrick, J. F.; Grindlay, J. H.; Mann, F. C.; and Deforest, R. E.: "Effect of Various Procedures on the Flow of Lymph," *Arch. Phys. Med.*, Vol. 34, No. 1, (Jan.) 1953, pp. 31–39.

Fulton, J. F.: *A Text Book of Physiology*, 16th ed. W. B. Saunders Co., Philadelphia, 1959.

Furscott, H. E.; Beard, B.; Rosman, G.; Elson, M.; and Anderson, M.: "Massage: Round Table and Demonstration," *Phys. Therapy Rev.*, Vol. 20:1, (Jan.-Feb.) 1940, pp. 29–41.

Gammon, G. D., and Starr, I.: "Studies on the Relief of Pain by Counter-irritation," *J. Clin. Invest.*, Vol. 20, No. 13, (Jan.) 1941.

Garrett, J. F.: *Psychological Aspects of Physical Disability*. Washington, D. C., U. S. Government Printing Office, Rehabilitation Service Series, No. 210, 1946.

Graham, D.: *Massage Manual Treatment and Remedial Movements*, 4th ed. J. B. Lippincott Co., Philadelphia, 1913.

Head, Sir Henry: *Studies in Neurology*. Henry Frowde and Hodder and Stoughton, London, 1920.

Hertzman, A.: "The Physiology and Measurement of Circulation," *Phys. Therapy Rev.*, Vol. 30, No. 11, (Nov.) 1950, pp. 471–81.

Hickey, H. K.: "A Kit of Tools," *Phys. Therapy Rev.*, Vol. 31, No. 4, (Apr.) 1951, pp. 135–38.

Hoffa, A. J.: *Technik der Massage,* 3rd ed. Ferdinand Enke, Verlagsbuchhandlung, Stuttgart, 1900.

Jacobs, Miriam: "Massage for the Relief of Pain: Anatomical and Physiological Considerations," *Phys. Therapy Rev.,* Vol. 40, No. 2, (Feb.) 1960, pp. 96–97.

Karnosh, L. J., and Mereness, D.: *Psychiatry for Nurses.* C. V. Mosby Co., St. Louis, 1944.

Kelly, H. T.: "Psychosomatic Aspects of Physical Medicine," *Phys. Therapy Rev.,* Vol. 28, No. 6, (Nov.-Dec.) 1948, pp. 280–83.

Kimber, Diana C.; Gray, Carolyn E.; Stackpole, Caroline E.; and Leavell, Lutie C.: *Textbook of Anatomy and Psysiology,* 14th ed. The Macmillan Company, New York, 1961.

Kleen, E. H. G.: *Massage and Medical Gymnastics,* 2nd ed. Williams and Wood Co., 1921.

Kosman, A. J.; Wood, E. C.; and Osborne, S. L.: "The Effect of Massage upon the Skeletal Muscle of the Dog," *Arch. Phys. Med.,* Vol. XXIX, No. 8, (Aug.) 1948, pp. 489–90.

Ladd, M. P.; Kottke, F. J.; and Blanchard, R. S.: "Studies of the Effect of Massage on the Flow of Lymph from the Foreleg of the Dog," *Arch. Phys. Med.,* Vol. XXXIII, No. 10, (Oct.) 1952, pp. 604–12.

Leube H., and Dicke, Elisabeth: *Massage Reflektorischer Zonen im Bindegewebe.* Gustav Fischer, Jena, 1948.

Licht, S.: *Massage, Manipulation and Traction.* Elizabeth Licht, New York, 1960.

Lloyd, D. P. C.: "Principles of Nervous Activity," Sec. I, *Textbook of Physiology* (edited by J. F. Fulton). W. B. Saunders Co., Philadelphia, 1955.

Ludwig, A. O.: "Emotional Factors in Rheumatoid Arthritis," *Phys. Therapy Rev.,* Vol. 29, No. 8, (Aug.) 1949, pp. 339–44.

MacKenzie, J.: *Angina Pectoris.* Henry Frowde and Hodder and Stoughton, London, 1923.

Mahoney, L.: "Massage of Reflex Zones," *Physiotherapy* (J. of the Chartered Society of Physiotherapy), Vol. 43, (Mar.) 1957, p. 74.

Martin, G., et al.: "Cutaneous Temperature of the Extremities of Normal Subjects and of Patients with Rheumatoid Arthritis,"

Part III "Effect of Massage on Peripheral Circulation of the Extremities," *Arch. Phys. Med.,* Vol. 27, No. 11, (Nov.) 1946, pp. 665–82.

Maslow, A. H., and Mittelmann, B.: *Principles of Abnormal Psychology.* Harper and Brothers, New York, 1941.

McMillan, Mary: *Massage and Therapeutic Exercise,* 3rd ed. W. B. Saunders Co., Philadelphia, 1932.

Mennell, J. B.: *Physical Treatment by Movement, Manipulation, and Massage,* 4th ed. The Blakiston Co., Philadelphia, 1940.

——————: *Massage: Its Principles and Practice.* The Blakiston Co., Philadelphia, 1920.

Nissen, H.: *Practical Massage and Corrective Exercises.* F. A. Davis Co., Philadelphia, 1939.

Pemberton, R.: "The Physiological Influence of Massage," *Principles and Practice of Physical Therapy,* Vol. I. W. F. Prior Co., Inc., 1937.

Pinter, R.; Eisenson, J.; and Stanton, Mildred: *The Psychology of the Physically Handicapped.* F. W. Crofts and Co., New York, 1941.

Pollock, L. J., et al.: "The Effect of Massage and Passive Movement upon the Residuals of Experimentally Produced Section of the Sciatic Nerves of the Cat," *Arch. Phys. Med.,* Vol. XXXI, No. 5, (May) 1950, pp. 265–76.

Scull, C. W.: "Massage—Physiologic Basis," *Arch. Phys. Med.,* Vol. 26, No. 3, (Mar.) 1945, pp. 159–67.

Smith, Lola E.: "Role of Physical Therapy in Care of Psychiatric Patients," *Phys. Therapy Rev.,* Vol. 31, No. 4, (Apr.) 1951, pp. 123–26.

Solomon, W. M.: "What is Happening to Massage?" *Arch. Phys. Med.,* Vol. 31, (Aug.) 1950, pp. 521–23.

Storms, H. D.: "Diagnostic and Therapeutic Massage," *Arch. Phys. Therapy,* Vol. XXV, (Sept.) 1944, pp. 550–52.

Suskind, M. I.; Hajek, N. M.; and Hine, H. M.: "Effects of Massage on Denervated Skeletal Muscle," *Arch. Phys. Med.,* Vol. 27, No. 133, (Mar.) 1946.

Tappan, Frances: "Modern Massage Technics" (Unpublished Master's Thesis). Stanford University, Stanford, California, 1948.

——————: "Trends in Modern Massage Technics," *Phys. Therapy Rev.*, Vol. 35, No. 10, (Oct.) 1955.

——————: "Usefulness of Massage," *Brit. J. Phys. Med.*, (Aug.) 1957, Butterworth and Co., London.

Tidy, N. M.: *Massage and Remedial Exercises,* 4th ed. Williams and Wilkins, Baltimore, 1939.

von Werssowetz, O. F.: "Psychiatric Rehabilitation of Brachialgia," *Phys. Therapy Rev.*, Vol. 32, No. 4, (Apr.) 1952, pp. 163–69.

Wakim, K. G.: "The Effects of Massage on the Circulation in Normal and Paralyzed Extremities," *Arch. Phys. Med.*, Vol. XXX, (Mar.) 1949, pp. 135–44.

Wolff, A.: "Bindegewebsmassage" (a mimeographed report). Elisabeth Dicke Institut, Uberlingen, 1956.

Wood, Elizabeth; Kosman, A. J.; and Osborne, S. L.: "Effects of Massage on Delaying Atrophy in Denervated Skeletal Muscle of the Dog," *Phys. Therapy Rev.*, Vol. 28, No. 6, (Nov.-Dec.) 1948, pp. 284–85.

Zausmer, Elizabeth: "Psychologic Implications in Poliomyelitis," *Phys. Therapy Rev.*, Vol. 30, No. 7, (July) 1950, pp. 259–63.

Index